NURTURING BONDS: A HOLISTIC GUIDE TO BREASTFEEDING BLISS

Nurturing Bonds: A Holistic Guide to Breastfeeding Bliss

Dr. Khushboo Gupta, Assistant Professor, Trilok Singh TT College, Lakshmangarh, Sikar, Rajasthan, India

A. Annapurna, Assistant Professor, Food Science and Nutrition, Sir Durga Malleswara Siddartha Mahila Kalasala, Vijayawada, India

Dr. Preeti Verma, Subject Matter Specialist (Home Science), Krishi Vigyan Kendra, Banasthali Vidyapith, Tonk, Rajasthan, India

Dr. Pratibha Pal, Assistant Professor, Home Science, Gandhi Satabdi Smarak P.G. College, Koilsa, Azamgarh, Uttar- Pradesh, India

Dr. Supriya, Senior Dietitian &HOD, Mediversal MultiSupar Speciality Hospital, Patna, Bihar, India

Hemakshee Publication

Nurturing Bonds: A Holistic Guide to Breastfeeding Bliss

Edition: 2024
ISBN: 978-81-969920-3-3

Published by Hemakshee Publication
Printed and Distributed by pothi.com

HEMAKSHEE PUBLICATION

Sikar, Rajasthan, India

publicationhemakshee@gmail.com

Website: hemaksheepublication.com

Contents

PREFACE

World breastfeeding week is a global campaign that aims to raise awareness and to promote breastfeeding as a vital component of maternal and infant health. It is celebrated from August 1st to august 7th every year and involves various events and activities organized by governments, non-government organization and communities worldwide. This week is celebrated in commemoration of the 1990 Innocenti declaration. World breastfeeding week started in year 1992, with annual themes including healthcare systems, women and work, the international code of marketing of breastmilk substitutes, community support, ecology, economy, science, education and human rights. Since year 2016, World breastfeeding week is aligned with sustainable development goals.

This week is celebrated every year with the objectives to raise awareness about the importance of breastfeeding for maternal and child health, nutrition and wellbeing; to advocate supportive policies and initiatives at the local, national and global levels to protect, promote and support breastfeeding; and to empower the mothers with information and support to make informed choices about breastfeeding.

Theme of year 2023 was **"Step up for breastfeeding - Educate and support"**. World breastfeeding week provides a platform for breastfeeding advocates, healthcare professionals, policymakers and communities to come together, share knowledge, experiences and work together creating a breastfeeding friendly world. It also serves as a reminder of the importance of supporting and protecting breastfeeding-friendly world. It also serves as a reminder of the importance of supporting and protecting breastfeeding for the health and wellbeing of mothers and infants.

Keeping this point of view "Jeevan Asheesh Sameeti", a non-profit organization from Kota city, Rajasthan and YouTube Channel "Dietitian Ki Salah" (an educational plateform for integrated health, wellness, wholesome nutrition, fitness and food) celebrated **'World Breastfeeding Week, 2023** and organized an essay writing competition for masses on various topics related to breastfeeding. People participated in this activity enthusiastically and appreciated the joint efforts of "Jeevan Asheesh Sameeti" and YouTube Channel "Dietitian Ki Salah" for this endeavour. Main aim of this activity was to aware common people about importance of breastfeeding for infants and lactating mothers, factors affecting breastfeeding, factors affecting breast milk supply and how the milk supply can be enhanced, etc. These topics are essential to improve quality of life of an infant and mothers as breastfeeding helps the mothers in dealing with postpartum depression, therefore, we are compiling those essays in the form of an edited book.

The edited book volume is primarily intended to be a collection of short chapters written by research scholars, academicians, doctors and faculty members of their respective fields. Chapters of this book entitled **"Nurturing Bonds: A Holistic Guide to Breastfeeding Bliss"** particularly based on topics such as importance of breastfeeding to child and mothers, nurturing our future, infant food, promote breastfeeding, lactation and solemnization of the bond of motherhood, importance of breastfeeding- a holistic approach, nourishing empowerment, the significance of breastfeeding: a comprehensive comparison with infant formula feeding, breastfeeding in special circumstances, breastfeeding support in India, a mother's journey through breastfeeding, etc.

We envisage the book to serve as a reference book for common people. This book will be very useful for students all over the globe, academicians, public health specialists, community science specialists, community development professionals, programmers of national and international agencies, and people of grass root level to aware them about different issues pertaining to acquire safe food and to maintain food security as well as libraries of relevant collages and institutions.

With great pleasure, we would like to extend our sincere thanks to all the authors of the chapters for reporting their thoughts and experience related to their work. We believe that this book is an important contribution to the community in addressing common issues pertaining to brain health and wellness.

It is our sincere hope that many more will join us in this time-critical endeavour and this book will stimulate discussions and generate helpful comments to improve future projects.

Happy reading and feedback awaited.

Dr. Khushboo Gupta
A. Annapurna
Dr. Preeti Verma
Dr. Pratibha Pal
Dr. Supriya

Introduction

Breastfeeding: Holistic Impact

Dr. Khushboo Gupta

Assistant Professor

Trilok Singh TT College

Lakshmangarh, Sikar (Rajasthan)

Email: drkhushboogupta2017@gmail.com

Introduction

Breastfeeding is a complex and multifaceted process that goes beyond the nourishment of a child. It encompasses psychological, social, physiological, and financial dimensions, impacting both the mother and child.

1. Psychological impact on mother and child

Breastfeeding initiates a powerful maternal bond, facilitated by the release of oxytocin, often referred to as the "love hormone." This emotional connection is not only vital for the infant's sense of security but also contributes significantly to the mother's mental well-being. Mothers who breastfeed may experience reduced rates of postpartum depression, attributed in part to hormonal changes during lactation.

Research suggests that the act of breastfeeding stimulates the release of dopamine, the pleasure neurotransmitter, reinforcing the positive emotional experience for both mother and child. Furthermore, the close physical contact during breastfeeding fosters a sense of comfort and security, laying the foundation for a strong parent-child relationship.

On the child's side, the psychological impact of breastfeeding extends beyond infancy. Studies indicate a potential link between breastfeeding and improved cognitive development, with breast milk containing essential nutrients and bioactive compounds that support neural growth. This aspect highlights the long-term benefits of the psychological connection established through breastfeeding.

2. Changes faced by mother and child

Physiological changes during breastfeeding are not confined to the mother's body; they extend to the child's development as well. For the mother, breastfeeding triggers the release of prolactin and oxytocin, hormones crucial for milk production and uterine contraction. This process aids in the recovery of the uterus postpartum and contributes to the natural spacing of pregnancies.

In contrast, the child experiences immediate physiological benefits from breastfeeding. Breast milk is a dynamic fluid that adapts to the changing needs of the infant. Colostrum, the first milk produced, is rich in antibodies, providing essential immune support during the vulnerable early days. As lactation progresses, the composition of breast milk adjusts to meet the nutritional requirements of the growing child, ensuring optimal development.

3. Psychological, social, and physiological factors

Breastfeeding has far-reaching implications for a mother's psychological well-being. The hormone oxytocin, released during breastfeeding, not only enhances maternal bonding but also acts as a natural stress-reliever. This hormonal response can contribute to a mother's overall mental health and emotional resilience, a crucial aspect of postpartum care.

Social support plays a pivotal role in the success of breastfeeding. Families, friends, and society at large influence a mother's decision and ability to breastfeed. A supportive environment can empower mothers, providing the encouragement and understanding needed to navigate potential challenges. Workplace policies that accommodate breastfeeding, such as dedicated lactation spaces and flexible schedules, contribute significantly to a positive social framework for breastfeeding mothers.

On a physiological level, breastfeeding offers numerous benefits. The composition of breast milk is finely tuned to the specific needs of the infant, providing not only essential nutrients but also immune factors that protect against infections. This dynamic adaptation reflects the biological synergy between mother and child, underscoring the innate physiological connection established through breastfeeding.

4. Financial factors associated with breastfeeding

The financial aspects of breastfeeding extend beyond the immediate costs of formula and feeding equipment. Breastfeeding can be more cost-effective than formula feeding in the long run. The absence of formula expenses, coupled with potential health benefits that may reduce medical costs, positions breastfeeding as a financially prudent choice for families.

Moreover, businesses and societies benefit from supporting breastfeeding mothers. Workplace policies that accommodate lactation needs, such as providing designated nursing spaces and flexible working hours, contribute to employee well-being. In turn, this support can enhance workplace morale, productivity, and employee retention, ultimately benefiting the financial bottom line.

5. Needs of mothers during lactation phase

Nutritional requirements during lactation demand attention to ensure both the mother and child receive adequate nourishment. Lactating mothers require additional calories, protein, and specific nutrients, emphasizing the importance of a well-balanced diet rich in vitamins and minerals. A comprehensive understanding of these nutritional needs is essential for promoting the health of both mother and child.

Support systems are critical for mothers during the lactation phase. Breastfeeding-friendly environments, both at home and in public spaces, help create a conducive atmosphere for nursing mothers. Workplace initiatives, such as providing comfortable lactation rooms and flexible schedules, play a pivotal role in addressing the needs of breastfeeding mothers, allowing them to balance work responsibilities with the demands of lactation.

6. Global perspectives on breastfeeding policies

Breastfeeding policies vary widely across the globe, influencing maternal choices and societal attitudes. In Scandinavian countries, for instance, extensive maternity leave and workplace accommodations contribute to high breastfeeding rates. Conversely, some regions face challenges due to insufficient policies and societal norms that may not fully support breastfeeding.

Investigating these global perspectives offers valuable insights into the effectiveness of different approaches. Comparing policies, cultural attitudes, and their impact on breastfeeding rates provides a nuanced understanding of how societal structures shape the breastfeeding experience.

7. Long-term health impacts

Beyond the immediate benefits, breastfeeding has lasting health implications for both mothers and children. Research suggests that mothers who breastfeed may experience a reduced risk of developing breast and ovarian cancers. Exploring these long-term health advantages emphasizes the importance of breastfeeding not only in the early stages of child development but also in promoting maternal health throughout a woman's life.

For children, the protective effects of breastfeeding extend to a decreased susceptibility to infections, allergies, and chronic conditions. Understanding these long-term health impacts highlights the significance of breastfeeding as a foundational element in building a healthier future generation.

8. Cultural influences on breastfeeding

Explore how cultural beliefs and practices impact breastfeeding. Different cultures may have unique perspectives on breastfeeding, affecting maternal choices and societal norms. Discussing cultural influences adds depth to the understanding of breastfeeding's broader context.

For instance, in some cultures, extended family involvement in childcare may influence breastfeeding practices, while in others, cultural perceptions of modesty and privacy can affect a mother's willingness to breastfeed in public. Recognizing and respecting these cultural variations is crucial for promoting inclusive and supportive environments for breastfeeding mothers globally.

9. Challenges and solutions

Address common challenges faced by breastfeeding mothers, such as lactation difficulties, societal stigmas, and balancing breastfeeding with work commitments. Provide practical solutions and support systems that can help overcome these challenges, promoting a realistic and positive portrayal of the breastfeeding journey.

Challenges may include inadequate workplace support, insufficient education on breastfeeding techniques, and societal pressures. Solutions can range from workplace policies that accommodate breastfeeding mothers to community-based support groups and educational initiatives to raise awareness about the benefits and challenges of breastfeeding.

10. Technological innovations and breastfeeding

In recent years, technological advancements have introduced various tools to support breastfeeding mothers. Breastfeeding apps, for example, offer features like tracking feeding schedules, monitoring infant growth, and providing educational resources. Smart breast pumps allow mothers to express milk efficiently, offering convenience and flexibility. Online support communities provide a platform for mothers to share experiences and seek advice. While these innovations can enhance the breastfeeding experience, it's essential to explore their impact on maternal confidence, mental well-being, and overall success in breastfeeding.

11. Environmental impact of infant formula production

The production and distribution of infant formula have significant environmental implications. The manufacturing process, packaging materials, and transportation contribute to a considerable carbon footprint. Contrasting this with breastfeeding, which requires no manufacturing or transportation, emphasizes the eco-friendly nature of breastfeeding. Discussing these environmental considerations adds a dimension to the conversation about infant nutrition, encouraging a broader perspective on sustainability in childcare practices.

12. Breastfeeding and public health

Breastfeeding plays a crucial role in public health by contributing to disease prevention. Studies have linked breastfeeding to a lower risk of respiratory and gastrointestinal infections in infants. Additionally, breastfeeding has been associated with a reduced risk of chronic conditions such as obesity and diabetes later in life. Understanding these public health implications underscores the importance of promoting breastfeeding as a preventive measure, potentially alleviating the strain on healthcare systems and improving long-term community health.

13. Breastfeeding and maternal employment

Employed mothers often face challenges when balancing breastfeeding with work responsibilities. Extended maternity leave, flexible working hours, and on-site childcare facilities can significantly impact a mother's ability to continue breastfeeding upon returning to work. Exploring the intersection of breastfeeding and maternal employment highlights the need for supportive workplace policies. Initiatives that accommodate lactation needs contribute not only to the well-being of mothers but also to a more inclusive and family-friendly work environment.

14. Myths and misconceptions surrounding breastfeeding

Addressing common myths and misconceptions about breastfeeding is essential for providing accurate information and support to mothers. Examples of myths include concerns about milk supply, the belief that formula is equivalent to breast milk, or misconceptions about the impact of breastfeeding on maternal physical appearance. Dispelling these myths with evidence-based information fosters a more informed and supportive community, empowering mothers to make confident and well-informed choices regarding breastfeeding.

15. Socioeconomic disparities in breastfeeding

Socioeconomic factors significantly influence breastfeeding practices, creating disparities that impact maternal and child health. Lower-income families may face barriers such as limited access to lactation consultants, shorter or nonexistent maternity leave, and financial constraints that make it challenging for mothers to exclusively breastfeed. Addressing these disparities involves advocating for policies that provide equal access to lactation resources, promoting workplace support for breastfeeding mothers, and ensuring that socioeconomic status does not hinder a mother's ability to make informed and supported choices regarding breastfeeding.

16.   Breastfeeding   and   infant   gut microbiome

Breast milk is not only a source of essential nutrients but also plays a crucial role in shaping the infant gut microbiome. The microbiome, a community of microorganisms in the digestive system, influences various aspects of health, including immune function and metabolism. Breast milk contains prebiotics that nourish beneficial bacteria and probiotics that actively contribute to the establishment of a healthy gut microbiome. Exploring this connection emphasizes the multifaceted benefits of breastfeeding beyond immediate nutrition, setting the foundation for the child's long-term well-being.

17. Breastfeeding in emergency situations

In emergency situations, breastfeeding becomes a lifeline for infants, providing a stable source of nutrition and immune support when access to clean water and formula may be compromised. Breast milk is readily available, requires no preparation, and reduces the risk of infections. Understanding the challenges faced by breastfeeding mothers in emergency situations, such as ensuring privacy and maintaining adequate nutrition, emphasizes the resilience of breastfeeding as a critical survival strategy for infants during times of crisis. Efforts to support breastfeeding in emergency settings can contribute to the overall well-being and survival of vulnerable populations.

18. Breastfeeding and Mental health

Explore the intricate relationship between breastfeeding and maternal mental health. While breastfeeding can contribute to emotional well-being through the release of oxytocin and the bonding experience, it's crucial to address the potential challenges. Some mothers may experience anxiety or stress related to breastfeeding, and societal expectations can contribute to feelings of guilt or inadequacy. Discussing the mental health aspects of breastfeeding promotes a holistic understanding, emphasizing the importance of providing emotional support and mental health resources for breastfeeding mothers.

19. Breastfeeding and allergies/ intolerances

Examine the role of breastfeeding in preventing or mitigating allergies and intolerances in infants. Breast milk contains antibodies and immune-boosting factors that may play a role in reducing the likelihood of allergic reactions. Understanding how breastfeeding contributes to the development of the infant immune system and its impact on allergies provides valuable insights into the broader health benefits associated with breastfeeding.

In conclusion, breastfeeding encompasses a rich tapestry of psychological, social, physiological, and financial dimensions. Exploring and addressing these multifaceted aspects can contribute to the well-being of both mothers and children, fostering a supportive environment that recognizes and accommodates the diverse needs associated with breastfeeding.

Understanding the complex interplay between breastfeeding and the development of allergies or intolerances provides valuable insights for healthcare professionals and mothers alike. While breastfeeding is not a guaranteed prevention method, its role in supporting the immune system and influencing the infant's tolerance to various foods underscores the multifaceted benefits of this natural feeding method.

Biography
(Dr. Khushboo Gupta)

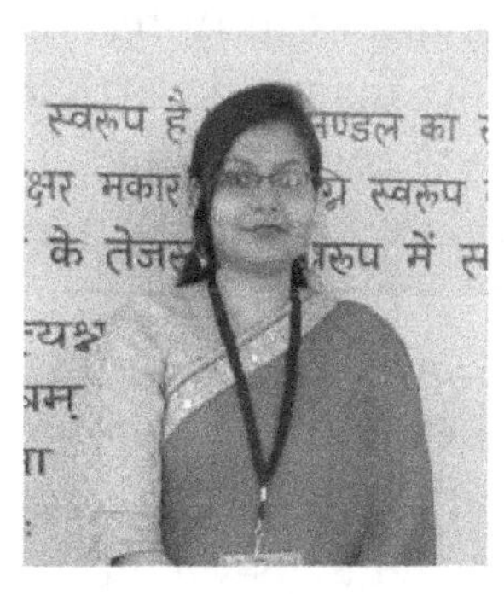

Dr. Khushboo Gupta is a PhD Home Science (Food Science and Nutrition) from Banasthali Vidyapith, Newai, India. She has been teaching subject including food chemistry, food analysis, therapeutic nutrition, human nutrition, human physiology and community nutrition, etc. Presently she is working as Assistant Professor in Trilok Singh TT College, Laxmangarh, Sikar, Rajasthan.

She is MSc Gold medalist and had **cleared UGC-NET and RPSC-SET examination.** Dr Gupta holds Advance Diploma in French Language from Banasthali Vidyapith; Diploma in Naturopathy and Yoga (NDDY) from Gandhi Smarak Prakritik Chikitsa Samiti (Regd.), New Delhi; Certificate in Homeopathic Medicinal System conducted by Vardhman Mahaveer Open University, Kota and Certificate in Statistical Techniques and Applications. She has featured in several programs of All India Radio and Radio Banasthali (FM 90.4).

Dr. Khushboo is actively involved in community activities especially those concerned with self-employment, health and wellness, optimum nutrition and how to improve quality of life of a person and family. She is the keynote speaker and founder of her YouTube channel "Dietitian Ki Salah" through which she provides education related to optimum health, wellness and nutrition to masses. Dr. Gupta has published about more than 30 research papers in reputed national and international journals; 7 book chapters in different edited books, several news paper and magazine articles related to health, nutrition and new food product formulation. She authored one book related to elderly nutrition; edited fifteen books related to community science, food science and nutrition, health and wellness, issues with girls, health for all, sustainable development, food safety and security, millets and handbook on IBD for upliftment of the individuals of the society. She presented her research work in more than 26 national and international conferences. Her research is primarily in the area of food processing entrepreneurial skill Inculcation and geriatric nutrition. **The patent office, Government of India has granted a patent to Dr. Khushboo for her research on food formulation using RSM.** Dr. Gupta has successfully completed more than 30 courses on various diverse topics organized by SWAYAM, UNICEF, WHO and Cornell University.

In past she had worked as Assistant Professor (Food and Nutrition) in Modi University, Laxmangarh, Sikar; worked as Master Trainer in Agriculture University, Kota. During her PhD she had worked as UGC- SRF in Banasthali Vidyapith, Newai. One feather in her cap is that she had worked as regular trainee dietitian in dietetics department of Post Graduate Institute of Medical Education and Research (PGIMER), Chandigarh and got her short-term attachment certificate. She won many awards in different seminars and conferences for her contribution in scientific world. Apart from them, she is rewarded with **Teacher Honour award** by Lions Club Kota South (September, 2017); '**Award of Honour**' given by All Rajasthan Qualified Homoeopathic Doctors Association in Homoeopathic Scientific Seminar, 2017 and **Excellence Academician Award** given by Akhil Bhartiya Agrawal Mahasabha (Reg), kota Branch (2023).

She is the life member of many reputed institutes i.e. Nutrition Society of India, Indian Dietetic Association, The Indian Science Congress Association and Institute of Scholars and giving her services for upliftment of community.

Biography
(A. Annapurna)

A. Annapurna is a research scholar, pursuing PhD in Food & Nutritional Sciences, Acharya Nagarjuna University. She has qualified UGC – NET for Asst. Professor, has 13 years of experience as a teaching faculty. She published research papers, participated in poster presentations, presented papers at 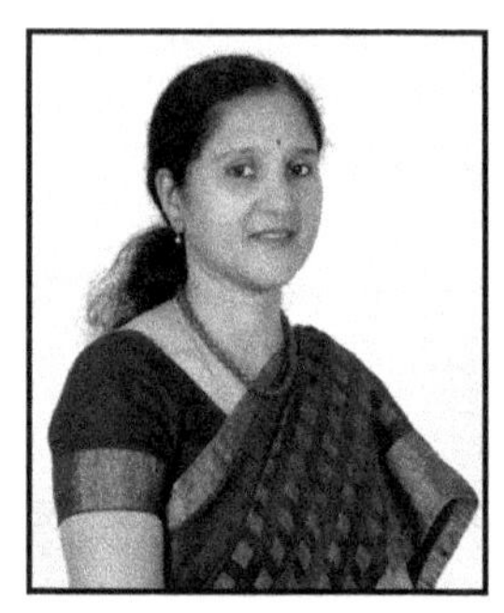 International Conferences and given guest lectures in colleges. She writes health articles, did YouTube videos and acts as a reviewer. She is adept at mentoring students –initiated YouTube channel, Food Doctor, published a booklet on Millets and helped in the direction of a street play 'Importance of Millets' by students. She addressed Anganwadi teachers in Poshan Pakwada 2023, ICDS Awareness Programme on 'Importance of Millets in Daily diets'. Apart from her academic pursuits she is interested in literary writing and authored three books – poetry, short stories and children's stories. She is currently working as Asst. Prof. (Food Science & Technology), working on her forthcoming books and is the Editor and Advisor of Muse India literary e-journal and Science Shore e-magazine. She received several accolades and awards. She was one of the delegates at the National Festival of Letters, 2023 and International Literary Festival – Unmesha (2023) conducted by Sahitya Akademi, Ministry of Culture.

Biography
(Dr. Preeti Verma)

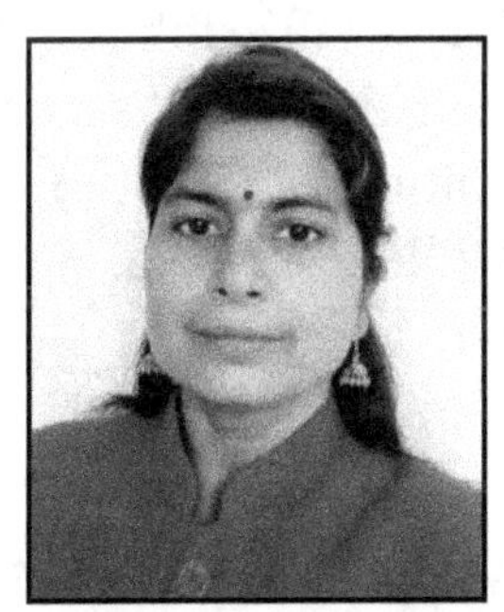

Dr Preeti Verma is a Subject Matter Specialist (Home Science) in Krishi Vigyan Kendra, Banasthali Vidyapith, Tonk, Rajasthan. She did her Ph.D. and M.Sc. from Banasthali Vidyapith, Rajasthan.

She also has given her services as Assistant Professor in the Department of Home Science, The IIS University, Jaipur, Rajasthan for 2.5 years and presently involved in research and extension activities in Krishi Vigyan Kendra since 2017. She has to her credit one book on preservation, two book chapters, thirty research papers in National and International Journals and seven popular articles in different magazines. She has actively participated and presented various research papers in National and International workshops, Seminars and conferences. She has also contributed to develop range of booklets, folders and study materials.

Biography
(Dr. Pratibha Pal)

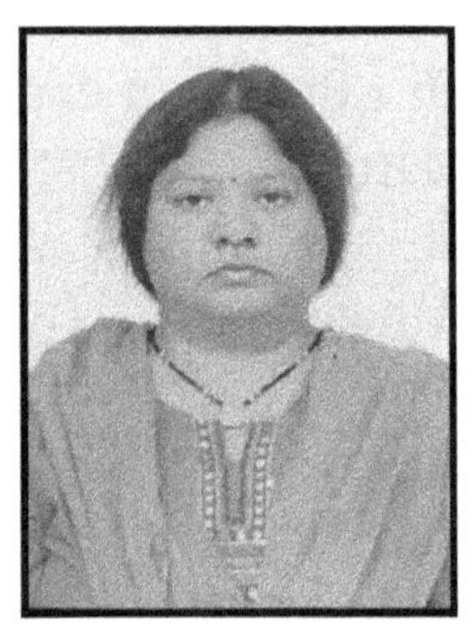

Dr. Pratibha Pal, currently working as Assistant Professor at Gandhi Satabdi Smarak P.G. College, Koilsa, Azamgarh, U.P. She is a professor with profound experience of teaching and research. She has completed her Ph.D in Home Science from CSJM University, Kanpur along with her Post Graduation in Home Science. She has completed her Bachelor Of Arts from Lucknow University in Home Science, Sociology and Anthropology. Her other degrees include B.Ed (Home Science, Social Science), M.Ed (Education) and Post Graduate Diploma in Information Technology.

She has the degree of UGC NET in Home Science. She is accented with the knowledge in the field of communication skill and soft skill to satisfy career in the field of teaching and research. She has published 25 International and 5 National research papers along with 3 Course books. She was highly active in various conferences (11), seminars (9), and workshops (5) in her time being. She has been awarded the "Young Scientist Award" by the SARSD New Delhi in 2021, "Excellent Academician Award" by ATDS, U.P. and "'Exellence Teaching Award" by ATDS, U.P.

Biography
(Dr. Supriya)

Dr. Supriya, PhD, MSc Food Science & Nutrition (RND, Sadhna Awardee 2024), Senior Dietitian, working as HOD, Dept. of Dietetics & Nutrition, Mediversal Multi Super Speciality Hospital, Patna, CDE, IYCF & Lactation Expert. About 10 years experience in the field of 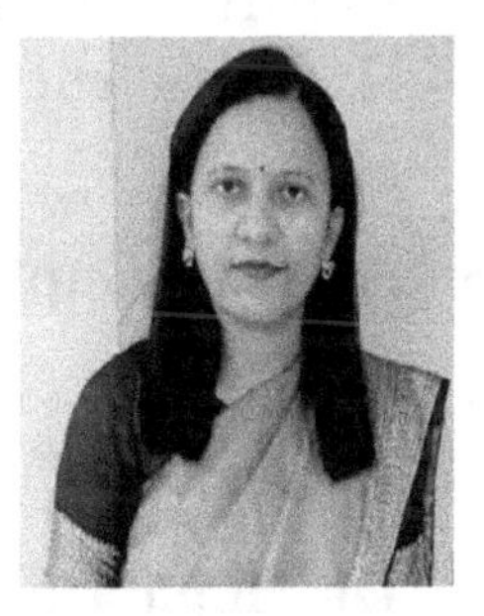 nutrition, research, public health & community nutrition as well. Invited as public health speaker, Keynote speaker, panelist, chairperson and organized various nutrition awareness camp, webinar, etc. Secretary IAPEN India Patna Chapter. Co-Convenor Netprofan Patna Chapter. She clear ESPEN (4 LLL exam in Lyon, France) 2023. She received Dietitian of the year award, ISSN International award. She presented papers in various national and international conferences. Several paper publication in national & International journals. She worked as facilitator/trainer for giving training to FD, staff nurse, medical pg students at CoE, NRC, Patna Medical College & Hospital. Live programme at DD Bihar on the occasion of world breast feeding week, 2019. Organizing committee member in various conference and seminar at Patna. Certified Diabetes Educator (NDEP IYCF Master training. Professional Membership of IDA, NSI, IAPEN, ISPEN, Netprofan, RSSDI.

List of Contributors

1. **Anthony Savio Herminio da Piedade Fernandes,** Founder Owner of Trading Equations, Goa, India

2. **Anupreet Kaur Sobti**, Ph.D. Research Scholar, Department of Foods and Nutrition, Government Home Science College, Chandigarh (Affiliated to Panjab University, Chandigarh), India

3. **Archana Gupta**, Homemaker, Kota, Rajasthan

4. **Dr Aditya R. Nimbkar**, M. S. (Obstetrics & Gynaecology)

5. **Dr Hena Dhir** (MD, MHA)Bachelor of Medicine and Bachelor of Surgery, Government Medical College, Patiala, India Master of Healthcare Administration, Loma Linda University, United States

6. **Dr Muzamil Nissar**, Institute of Home science Kashmir University, Hazratbal Srinagar, Jammu and Kashmir, India

7. **Dr. Anjali Juyal**, CCAS,MPUAT, Department of Resource Management and Consumer Science, Udaipur

8. **Dr. Chetna Rochani**, MD (Hom), PG-FHPC, N.D.D.Y. Consulting Homoeopathic Physician, Vadodara, Gujarat; Associate Professor & HOD, Department of Pathology P P Savani University, Kosamba, Surat.

9. **Dr. Pratibha S. Katkar**, Head and Asst. Prof., (Department of Home Economics), Yeshwant Mahavidyalaya, Wardha

10. **Dr. Ritu Pradhan**, Head and Associate Professor Department of Foods and Nutrition, Government Home Science College, Chandigarh (Affiliated to Panjab University, Chandigarh), India

11. **Dr. Samina M. Ausvi**, Professor, Community Medicine, Viswabharathi Medical College, Kurnool, Andhra Pradesh

12. **Dr. Tripti Tiwari**, Assistant Professor (Department of Home Science) , Jananayak Chandrashekhar University, Ballia (U.P.)

13. **Dr. Uzma Mustaq**, Researcher, Institute of Home science, University of Kashmir Hazratbal Srinagar, Jammu and Kashmir, India

14. **Ms Patricia Michael**, Assistant Professor, Department of Nutrition, St. Francis College for Women, Hyderabad, Telangana India

15. **Ms. Ifrah Rehman**, Assistant Professor, Department of Environmental Studies, Miranda House, University of Delhi

16. **Pooja R Singhania**, PhD (Food Science & Nutrition) Certified Infant & Young Child Feeding Counseling Specialist by BPNI, Certified MIYCN expert by IIT Mumbai, Founder, Nourish 1000 Days

17. **Surbhee Gupta**, Assistant at LIC of India

1.

Nourishing Empowerment: The Multifaceted Impact of Breastfeeding on Women's Strength and Identity

Dr Muzamil Nissar

Institute of Home science Kashmir University, Hazratbal Srinagar, Jammu and Kashmir, India

Breastfeeding has emerged as a pivotal aspect of maternal care, profoundly influencing both infant health and women's empowerment (Smith et al., 2018). Scientific literature consistently emphasizes its role in providing optimal nutrition and immune support for infants (Brown, 2017), establishing breastfeeding as a critical component in the early stages of human development (Jones & Brown, 2019). Across cultures, it assumes varied symbolic meanings, intertwining with rituals and traditions that highlight its cultural significance (Adams & Taylor, 2020).

The nutritional benefits of breastfeeding are well-documented, with breast milk recognized as the high standard for infant nutrition (Smith et al., 2018). Its composition, tailored to meet the evolving needs of the growing infant, provides essential nutrients and antibodies crucial for immune system development (Brown, 2017). Breastfeeding, therefore, stands as a powerful tool for ensuring the health and well-being of the next generation (Jones & Brown, 2019). Historically, breastfeeding has been ingrained in human societies, playing aimportant role in early survival and shaping societal structures (Adams & Taylor, 2020). From ancient civilizations to modern times, it has been a common thread weaving through the narrative of maternal care and infant nourishment, reinforcing its status as a timeless practice deeply rooted in human existence (Smith et al., 2018).

Culturally, breastfeeding takes on a multitude of meanings, serving as a vehicle for transmitting values and traditions from one generation to the next (Brown, 2017). Rituals surrounding breastfeeding reflect societal norms, reinforcing the interconnectedness of motherhood with broader cultural identity. The act of breastfeeding becomes a shared experience, contributing to a collective sense of community and continuity (Jones & Brown, 2019).Beyond its biological and cultural dimensions, breastfeeding holds a unique power in empowering women. The act of nursing establishes an intimate bond between mother and child, fostering emotional connections beyond the physical act of feeding (Adams & Taylor, 2020). This profound connection reinforces the maternal role as a source of life and strength, contributing to empowerment that transcends biological functions.

In addition to emotional empowerment, breastfeeding contributes to the physical well-being of mothers. Research indicates that breastfeeding is associated with numerous health benefits for women, including a reduced risk of certain cancers and enhanced postpartum recovery (Smith et al., 2018). This dual impact positions breastfeeding as a comprehensive strategy for promoting the well-being of the entire family unit (Brown, 2017).

Economically, breastfeeding presents advantages for women and families. The cost savings compared to formula feeding empower women to make informed choices aligned with their financial circumstances (Jones & Brown, 2019). This economic dimension adds another layer to the empowering aspects of breastfeeding, enabling women to navigate motherhood within the context of their broader socioeconomic realities.

In the face of societal norms and evolving cultural attitudes, breastfeeding becomes a vehicle for challenging and reshaping perceptions of women's roles. By embracing breastfeeding, women challenge stereotypes and reclaim agency over their bodies and maternal identities (Adams & Taylor, 2020), contributing to the broader discourse on gender roles and women's empowerment.

In conclusion, breastfeeding emerges as a multifaceted empowerment tool for women, encompassing biological, cultural, emotional, economic, and societal dimensions. Its historical continuity, cultural significance, and impact on maternal and infant health underscore its centrality in shaping the narrative of women's strength and identity. As we navigate modern motherhood, understanding and appreciating the empowering aspects of breastfeeding become essential for fostering a holistic approach to maternal care.

References

1. Smith, J., et al. (2018). Breastfeeding and Child Development: A Comprehensive Review.
2. Brown, A. (2017). Infant Sleep and Night Feeding Patterns During Later Infancy: Association with Breastfeeding Frequency, Daytime Duration, and Maternal Partnered Status.
3. Jones, L. R., & Brown, A. (2019). The experiences of breastfeeding for women with polycystic ovary syndrome: A qualitative study.
4. Adams, C., & Taylor, M. (2020). Cultural Meanings and Practices of Breastfeeding among Latina Mothers in the United States.

2.

Importance of Breast Feeding to Child and Mother

Anthony Savio Herminio da Piedade Fernandes

Founder Owner of Trading Equations, Goa

Email: anthonyfernandes9@gmail.com

1. Benefits of breastfeeding for the child's health and development

Breastfeeding offers an array of benefits for a child's health and development, establishing a strong foundation for their future well-being. Firstly, breast milk contains essential nutrients that are easily digestible and perfectly tailored to meet the infant's nutritional needs. It provides antibodies and immune factors that help protect against infections, reducing the risk of respiratory illnesses, ear infections, and gastrointestinal disorders. Furthermore, breastfeeding promotes healthy weight gain in infants, lowering the likelihood of obesity later in life. In addition to physical health benefits, breastfeeding positively impacts a child's cognitive development. The skin-to-skin contact during nursing enhances bonding between mother and baby while stimulating brain development through sensory experiences.

Breastfeeding has also been associated with improved cognitive performance and enhanced emotional intelligence in children. Ultimately, the advantages of breastfeeding extend beyond infancy as well. Breastfed children tend to have lower rates of chronic diseases such as diabetes, asthma, and certain cancers later in life.

2. The physical and emotional benefits of breastfeeding for the mother

Breastfeeding not only provides numerous benefits for the child but also offers significant advantages to the mother's physical and emotional well-being. Physically, breastfeeding helps mothers recover from childbirth more quickly by stimulating the uterus to contract, reducing postpartum bleeding and aiding in weight loss. It also lowers the risk of developing certain types of cancers, including breast and ovarian cancer. Moreover, breastfeeding promotes a strong emotional bond between mother and child. The release of oxytocin during breastfeeding creates feelings of love and affection, fostering a deep connection that enhances maternal confidence and nurtures a positive maternal-infant relationship. This emotional bonding can alleviate stress levels in new mothers, reduce the risk of postpartum depression, and enhance overall mental health.

3. Breastfeeding: a bonding experience between mother and child

Breastfeeding is not merely a means of providing nourishment to an infant; it is a profound bonding experience that creates an unbreakable connection between a mother and her child. The physical closeness and skin-to-skin contact during breastfeeding promote feelings of warmth, comfort, and security for both mother and baby. During this intimate act, the mother's body releases hormones such as oxytocin, often referred to as the "love hormone." This hormone not only stimulates milk production but also fosters a deep emotional bond between mother and child. As the baby suckles at their mother's breast, they feel safe, loved, and protected. Moreover, breastfeeding establishes a unique form of communication between mother and child. Through breastfeeding cues like rooting or hand movements, the baby signals their hunger or need for comfort.

4. Overcoming challenges: promoting and supporting breastfeeding

Breastfeeding is a natural and essential process that provides numerous benefits for both the child and mother. However, despite its importance, many women face challenges when it comes to initiating and maintaining breastfeeding. To ensure successful breastfeeding outcomes, it is crucial to address these challenges by promoting and supporting this practice. One significant challenge faced by mothers is a lack of knowledge about breastfeeding techniques and its benefits. Providing comprehensive education during prenatal classes and through community health programs can empower women with the necessary information, boosting their confidence in breastfeeding. Additionally, societal barriers such as limited workplace support and inadequate maternity leave policies hinder mothers from continuing exclusive breastfeeding. Employers should implement supportive measures like designated lactation spaces, flexible work schedules, and extended maternity leave to enable mothers to breastfeed successfully.

Furthermore, addressing common concerns such as low milk supply or difficulty latching can be achieved through accessible lactation consultants or support groups.

3.

Importance of Breastfeeding as Infant Food

Dr. Tripti Tiwari

Assistant Professor (Department of Home Science)

Jananayak Chandrashekhar University, Ballia (U.P.)

Abstract

Breastfeeding is very important in the form of infant's diet - Mother's milk - Mother's milk is considered to be the best and natural food of the child. For a few months after birth, the child should get only mother's milk. Breastfeeding enhances the physical beauty of the mother, because when the baby drinks milk, the muscles of the breasts contract rapidly and take their natural form. Mother's milk contains all the nutrients in proper quantity for the growth and development of the child, such as carbohydrates, water, fat, vitamins, mineral salts, etc. After the birth of the child, a simple substance comes for three to four days. This simple substance is very essential for the growth and development of the child. This is called colostrum. Colostrum is a clear yellow colored substance. Protein content and vitamins in colostrum quantity is found. It is digestible.

Method of breastfeeding

While breastfeeding, both the mother and the child should be in a comfortable position. For this, the mother should sit comfortably taking the child in her lap with her left hand. The left hand should be placed under the child's head. The nipple should be given to the baby's mouth with the right hand. Hold the nipple with the hand in such a way that the baby can breathe easily. Before breastfeeding the child, the mother should wash her nipples with warm water and soap, so that sweat and dirt cannot be sucked by the child. If the baby is not in a comfortable position, he will not be able to drink the full amount of milk.

The mother should not give her milk every time the baby cries. Digestion is not regular in this. Children should be given milk at an interval of 3-3 hours. The child asks for milk from time to time too, but within a short period of time the time for drinking his milk becomes fixed. The child should be given milk during the day. The time of milk of the baby is as follows: 3 times in the morning, 6 o'clock, 9 o'clock, 12 o'clock in the afternoon, evening, morning and afternoon, the baby should be fed milk for 5 minutes. As the baby grows, the time of feeding should be increased. Gradually the baby can be fed milk for 8-10 minutes. Every time the child should be fed milk from both the sides. 6 o'clock at 9 o'clock.

Patting - While drinking milk, some air also enters the baby's stomach along with the milk. That air causes pain in the stomach of the child. The child should be patted slowly by touching the shoulder, so that he may belch and the air in the stomach comes out. There is no fear of vomiting even by stroking the child. That's why the baby must be patted after feeding. As a baby food, the health of the baby depends on a balanced diet. Proper diet is necessary for the physical growth and development of the child. The loss of energy due to the child's playing and jumping is made up for by diet only.

Human milk is the best natural food for babies. It can reduce infectious morbidity and mortality in infants and children and reduce the risk of childhood overweight and obesity during both childhood and adulthood. Women who breastfeed are less likely to develop breast and ovarian cancer in later life. They are also protected from the development of cancer and diabetes. The World Health Organization (WHO) recommends that breastfeeding should begin within one hour of birth and continue for up to 6 months without additional water, other liquids, or solids. In addition, WHO has set a target to achieve Exclusive Breastfeeding (EBF) rate. 50 percent for all infants under 6 months of age by 2025. However, currently, only about 42% of babies worldwide are breastfed within the first hour after birth and 41% are between 0 and 6 months, data from 2013-2018 show. Babies of 6 months are exclusively breastfed.

Mother's milk is like nectar for the baby. Breast milk contains essential nutrients, minerals, vitamins, proteins, fats, antibodies and immune factors that are essential for the overall development and health of the newborn. Up to six months after the birth of the baby, the mother's milk alone fulfills all the needs of the complete diet for the baby. Breastfeeding is beneficial for both the mother and the baby.

Benefits of breastfeeding to the baby

- Mother's milk contains all the nutrients, which are essential for the overall development of the baby. Mother's milk is considered a complete diet for the child.

- Breast milk contains high proteins and antibodies which boost the immunity of the baby.

- Mother's milk is manufactured according to the digestive system of the baby and the nutrients present in the mother's milk are easily digestible, which the baby can easily digest.

- DHA in mother's milk This happens, due to which the vision of the child also becomes sharp.

- Breastfeeding provides probiotics, which help fight infections in the baby's digestive system and keep the baby's digestive system healthy and less prone to stomach problems.

- Breastfeeding helps reduce the risk of Sudden Infant Death Syndrome.

- Colostrum, rich in Vitamin A and antibodies, helps in development by adapting to the needs of the newborn. Proteins, vitamins, calcium etc. present in mother's milk help in the physical development of the baby.

- Breast milk contains longchain polyunsaturated fatty acids, which play an important role in the mental development of the baby.

- Mother's milk is 100% safe, so there is less chance of allergies in breastfed babies, whereas other types of milk can be prone to allergies.

- There is no deficiency of proteins and vitamins in the body of the infant by breastfeeding and the calcium present in the mother's milk is absorbed by the baby, which works to strengthen the bones.

Benefits of breastfeeding to mother

- Breastfeeding reduces the risk of breast and ovarian cancer.

- Breastfeeding enhances and strengthens the emotional bond between mother and child.

- Breastfeeding helps in reducing weight, when a mother breastfeeds her baby, her body burns around 450 to 500 calories, it helps in reducing weight naturally.

A lactating mother must have a balanced diet rich in nutrients. A lactating mother should take special care of her diet because whatever she eats during this time affects her baby. There are certain foods that specifically help increase milk production; such foods are known as galactagogues.

4.

Nurturing Our Future: Exploring the Interplay between Breastfeeding and Sustainability

Ms. Ifrah Rehman

Assistant Professor,

Department of Environmental Studies, Miranda House, University of Delhi

Email:ifrah,rehman05@gmail.com

Abstract

This paper delves into the intricate relationship between breastfeeding and sustainability, examining how the practice of breastfeeding can contribute to a more sustainable future. Since the focus on this topic has been low, this paper explores the multifaceted connections between breastfeeding, environmental conservation, health, and social well-being. By analysing existing literature and drawing on interdisciplinary perspectives, this paper aims to shed light on the potential of breastfeeding as a tool for promoting sustainable development and fostering a harmonious relationship between human societies and the planet.

Introduction

The global pursuit of sustainability necessitates a holistic approach that encompasses environmental, social, and economic considerations. Breastfeeding, a natural and time-tested method of nourishing infants, emerges as a topic of relevance within the sustainability discourse due to its potential to impact multiple dimensions of well-being. This paper seeks to explore the intersections between breastfeeding and sustainability, highlighting the ways in which this maternal practice can contribute to the achievement of global sustainability goals. This paper examines the life and considers the experiences of breastfeeding women: both new-age moms and old mothers and tries to analyse the natural process from a fresh lens of conservation and sustainable development/sustainability. Promoting and facilitating breastfeeding tends to fulfil eleven out of the seventeen SDGs for the nations.

Breastfeeding and environmental sustainability

Formula feeding which became popular as recently as 100 years ago, has a notable environmental impact due to the resources required for manufacturing, packaging, and distributing infant formula. It requires a significant amount of water for its production, 4000 litres of water to produce 1 kg of infant formula powder. It has massive energy consumption and the production leads to emission of Green House Gases (GHGs). The packaging is made up of plastic, mostly single-use. Annually over 400,000 tonnes of plastic waste from formula packaging end up in landfills. This waste along with food waste can take years to decompose and harms the wildlife and ecosystems. The carbon footprint from transportation also varies widely. The production ingredients such as dairy and soy requires agricultural land leading to deforestation, habitat loss, agricultural run-off, impacting local ecosystems.

Breastfeeding, unlike formula feeding, generates minimal environmental impact. It requires no packaging, reduces energy consumption, and conserves natural resources. This section examines the environmental benefits of breastfeeding emphasising its role in mitigating climate change and promoting ecological balance. The production and distribution of formula requires significant amount of water and energy consumption while breastfeeding relies on the body's natural processes without the need for manufacturing, transportation, and packaging, thereby reducing the generation of plastic waste associated with formula containers and packets.

It is produced on-demand and does not lead to food waste unlike packaged formula that might be discarded if not consumed within a specific time frame. Breastfeeding eliminated the need for resource intensive production processes. Thus, it promotes biodiversity and leads to less chemical exposure for infants enhancing their overall health.

Breastfeeding emits 20-50 times less CO_2 equivalent emissions than formula feeding due to the reduced energy and resource requirements

Breastfeeding also contributes to healthier infants with fewer medical interventions as per health and dietary experts. This reduces healthcare related waste and the associated carbon emissions from the healthcare facilities.

Breastfeeding and public health

Breastfeeding is closely linked to improved infant and maternal health outcomes. Breast milk provides essential nutrients, antibodies, and enzymes that bolster a child's immune system and promote healthy growth. This section delves into the long-term implications of breastfeeding on public health, including its potential to reduce healthcare costs, enhance food security, and contribute to healthier populations.

On infant health

Breastfeeding leads to **reduced mortality and morbidity** – According to UNICEF and a study published in The Lancet which estimated that optimal breastfeeding practices could prevent around 800,000 child deaths per year from pneumonia and diarrhoea. Breastfed infants have 14 times lower risk of dying in the first six months compared to non-breastfed infants.

Reduced infections – Breastmilk provides essential antibodies and immune factors. Exclusive breastfeeding for the first six months reduces the risk of common childhood infections, including respiratory and gastrointestinal infections.

Cognitive development – A meta-analysis published in the American Journal of Clinical Nutrition showed that breastfeeding is associated with a 15-30% reduction in the risk of childhood obesity.

On maternal health

Postpartum weight loss - Women who breastfeed tend to lose pregnancy weight more effectively. A study published in the American Journal of Clinical Nutrition found that women who exclusively breastfed for at least three months had greater postpartum weight loss compared to non-breastfeeding mothers.

Reduced risk of breast cancer - A meta-analysis published in The Lancet estimated that breastfeeding could prevent approximately 20,000 breast cancer cases per year worldwide.

Ovarian Cancer and Type 2 Diabetes Prevention - The Nurses' Health Study found that longer duration of breastfeeding was associated with a lower risk of developing type 2 diabetes as well as reduced risk of ovarian cancer.

Maternal Mental Health - A study published in the International Journal of Obstetrics and Gynaecology found that breastfeeding for at least two months was associated with a lower risk of postpartum depression.

Challenges and Considerations

While breastfeeding aligns with sustainability ideals, various challenges hinder its widespread adoption. Societal attitudes, workplace policies, and inadequate support systems can discourage mothers from breastfeeding. This paper gives a semblance of facts in order to address those challenges and highlights the importance of creating an enabling environment for breastfeeding through policy initiatives, workplace accommodations, and public awareness campaigns.

Education and advocacy play a pivotal role in promoting breastfeeding as a sustainable practice. More efforts will prove the significance of raising awareness about the environmental, health, and societal benefits of breastfeeding. It also emphasizes the need for interdisciplinary collaboration among healthcare professionals, environmentalists, policymakers, and activists to drive positive change.

Conclusions

Breastfeeding emerges as a powerful nexus between maternal instinct, infant health, environmental stewardship, and societal well-being. This paper underscores the multifaceted contributions of breastfeeding to sustainability. It calls for concerted efforts to integrate breastfeeding promotion into broader sustainability agendas, thereby nurturing future generations while fostering a harmonious relationship with the planet. By recognizing the inherent sustainability of breastfeeding and working collectively to overcome obstacles, societies can harness this natural practice to create a more sustainable and prosperous future for all. As one participant for this research said, "Babies are expensive. The only thing free, convenient, healthy and easily accessible is breastmilk."

5.

Breastfeeding - A Community Responsibility

Dr. Samina M. Ausvi

Professor, Community Medicine,

Viswabharathi Medical College, Kurnool, Andhra Pradesh

Mrs Anitha, a labourer who stopped breastfeeding after 4 months as she had to return to her work to earn livelihood. If we look around us carefully, so many women with different reasons for early cessation of breastfeeding are there. The question arises; Who is responsible for it? Is it the woman, her family, community or policies? Breast milk is perfectly adapted to the needs of the infant containing adequate amount of proteins, fats, carbohydrates and minerals in easily digestible form. Milk proteins help in the growth, building immunity and in protection of infants against infectious diseases. Colostrum is also called as first vaccine for newborn. Breastfeeding is the most cost effective intervention which saves lives, improves health, and contributes to social and economic development of community and nation. Breastfeeding prevents diseases and deaths in children and breast and ovarian cancer in mothers. Early initiation of breastfeeding within an hour of birth recommended by

WHO, can prevent neonatal mortality; whereas exclusive breastfeeding for six months significantly reduces episodes of diarrhoea and pneumonia in infants and young children.NFHS-5 data of India revealed that children under age of 3 years breastfed within one hour of birth are 41.8 % and children under the age of 6 months exclusively breastfed are 54.9% with less percentage in rural than in urban areas. There is a need of research in this to deepen the understanding of disparities in breastfeeding initiation, duration, continuation and the roles of other stakeholders in supporting breastfeeding.

Embracing motherhood is a challenge; many women are not prepared for it so they feel nervous and anxious. Many mothers encounter various barriers to breastfeeding which are not in their control. These can be at social, cultural, economical and political level. Sometimes there will be primary physiological inability to breastfeed like polycystic ovary syndrome, hypoplastic breasts and rarely woman on drugs which are contraindicated with breastfeeding and postnatal depression. Sometimes neonatal conditions like cleft lip and cleft palate or tongue tie are also the affecting factors. There are many reasons why women avoid or stop breastfeeding. It ranges from the medical, cultural and psychological to physical discomfort and inconvenience. Many times trivial reasons make mothers to adopt formula feeding. Issues with stretched professional care, negative social attitudes, body image, low maternal self efficacy, conflicting responsibilities and a lack of familial and community support act as barriers to breastfeeding. Lacking access to health care resources leads to inadequate knowledge about tackling the issues related to breastfeeding.

We can't always blame mother for failure of breastfeeding. Breastfeeding is not a closed-loop between mothers and babies but it is an experience and responsibility that must be shared. It should be shared by the partner, family, community and the government. Though individual support is important, breastfeeding must be considered a public health issue that requires efforts at community level. Promotive, preventive, public health approach and interventions at different health care levels to empower women to breastfed is a need of hour. Measures to resolve social, economic and political issues which influence the knowledge, attitudes and ability to make appropriate breastfeeding decisions should be undertaken. On a policy level, it should involves prioritising breastfeeding, with increased resources needed for health care providers to spend more time with new mothers during pregnancy, labour and postnatal period.

Measures which should be undertaken to improve breastfeeding initiation and continuation rates can be broadly divided under following five broad categories.

1. Care during antenatal, intranatal and postnatal period

Maternal experiences during antenatal, intranatal and post-natal care have impact upon breastfeeding attitudes and practices at both a physiological and psychological level. Many breastfeeding issues can be prevented if women had better knowledge, healthy environment and extended support. Starting from antenatal period, high-quality detailed antenatal breastfeeding education by well qualified and trained health care personnel is needed. It should be focused on the realities and challenges breastfeeding rather than aiming to increase intention alone. Breastfeeding education highlighting the benefits of breastfeeding to mother, child, family and community as well as discussing the process of breastfeeding and how it differ from formula feeding should be included. Fathers also play an important role in supporting mothers emotionally and in decision-making so they should also be the part of antenatal breastfeeding education and counselling sessions. In caesarean section delivery, there will be associated pain, the release of oxytocin and prolactin is weaker, delayed milk production which eventually leads to delayed breastfeeding.

Medications during labour, particularly pethidine if used, can also affect breastfeeding outcomes because of sub optimal rooting and latch. Epidural anaesthesia has also been associated with reduced breastfeeding continuation. Hospitals which are accredited under Baby Friendly Hospital Initiative which follows all the steps to successful breastfeeding have higher breastfeeding rates. Rooming-in and skin-to-skin contact of baby provides warmth and improves mother child bond helping in successful breastfeeding.

2. Family support

Mothers, fathers, grandmothers or any other family member who accompanies nursing mothers should be equipped to understand the importance of breastfeeding and its benefits for the health and development of the child; Peer support groups offer an additional level to this. The attitudes and experiences of those close to the mother do matter. These people should be updated on current guidelines on breastfeeding. Grandmothers/mothers-in-law should also be targeted because they can pass on their positive or negative experiences, practical advice which can influence breastfeeding decision-making in new mothers.

Utmost importance should be given to protect and promote mother's health. Providing her with good quality food rich in calories, proteins, calcium and other micronutrients should be made available and accessible for every nursing woman is a responsibility of a family and community.

3. Work place support

Employers must provide mothers with the necessary means to continue breastfeeding like access to paid maternity and paternity leaves which is associated with longer breastfeeding duration. On return to work, provide a room for mothers to be able to breastfeed.

4. National laws & policy

Policy and law to protect the dignity of breastfeeding mothers should be developed. Breastfeeding should not be viewed as provocative and safe places for breastfeeding should be made available at work places, transport terminals, cafes, restaurants and public places. National laws should stringently regulate the large-scale promotion of breast milk substitutes in order to protect breastfeeding.

5. Breastfeeding promotional activities

The activities advocating methods and advantages of breastfeeding should not be limited to only for a week in August. Wider public health campaigns to improve public perceptions of breastfeeding should be conducted throughout the year. Breast feeding and its benefits should be added as a social education in school curriculum so that at younger age only students will understand its importance and will be able to deal with challenges in later life.

Gynaecologists, Paediatricians, nurses, doctors, and all other health care providers should engage in the promotion of breastfeeding and work to create a favourable environment in health institutions and local communities through health education. Effective implementation of a nationwide programme like - 'MAA' (Mothers' Absolute Affection) which involves a comprehensive set of activities on promotion and support of breastfeeding at community and facility levels, through building an enabling environment reinforcing lactation support services at public health facilities through trained healthcare providers and awareness generation activities at community level is required.

Support offered for breastfeeding at family and community level, determines the maternal decision making related to breastfeeding. All the barriers like physical, psychological, economic, social, cultural and political should be dealt with government investment in promotional strategies of breastfeeding through trained health care providers. Improving knowledge, perceptions and practices related to breastfeeding through supportive environment is the key to sustain breastfeeding. Targeting the whole community for promotional activities rather than mothers only and individualized one-to-one support for lactating woman is vital.

6.

Importance of Breastfeeding: A Holistic Approach

Dr Hena Dhir (MD, MHA)

Bachelor of Medicine and Bachelor of Surgery, Government Medical College, Patiala, India

Master of Healthcare Administration, Loma Linda University, United States

Breast feeding is an ancient practice that has gained worldwide recognition and appreciation for its crucial role in the establishment of health for infants and mothers. It provides a plethora of nutritional advantages for the baby and promotes excellent health outcomes for both the baby and the mother. The health benefits of breastfeeding extend beyond infancy, with breastfed children exhibiting lower susceptibility to infections, allergies, and chronic diseases later in life. The presence of protective antibodies in breast milk contributes to a robust immune system, reducing the likelihood of common childhood ailments.

These innumerable advantages of breast milk are not just limited to babies but also extend to mothers. Breastfeeding promotes post-partum recovery for the mother by facilitating the reduction of uterine size to its pre pregnancy state. It minimizes the risk of bleeding after the birth of the child and reduces the mother's risk of high blood pressure, type 2 DM, ovarian cancer, and breast cancer. Not only this, but breast feeding also promotes attachment between mother and her baby, thereby creating a calming, relaxing and stress relieving environment for maternal child bonding. This mitigates the risk for post- partum depression and promotes the overall well- being of the mother and her child.

Given the multitude of advantages that breast feeding has to offer, certain work life scenarios can make it difficult for working mothers to balance work and maternal- child time thereby increasing anxiety and uneasiness. To address this issue, workplaces must adopt supportive policies and practices. Establishing lactation rooms, implementing flexible work schedules, and offering remote work options can accommodate the breastfeeding needs of working mothers. Paid maternity leave policies are essential to allow mothers sufficient time to establish breastfeeding routines without compromising their financial stability. It is extremely crucial to relax while nursing. Stress can create a detrimental impact on milk production and release. Therefore, it is crucial for lactating mothers to take their time to acclimatize themselves to creating a work-life balance and breastfeed effectively. In case the mother wishes to use a breast pump at work, she must ensure that she has all the means to pump, collect, store and transport the breast milk. This will include milk storage bags, cooler bag for transporting the milk, nursing pads and spare clothing in case of milk leakage. The best times to pump milk should coincide with the times that the mother would normally breast feed her baby. The expressed milk can be kept chilled in a fridge. Since the milk is kept chilled in fridge and transported home via a cooler bag, it is safe for child's consumption for 2-3 days. To promote this practice effectively, employer education programs should be offered to create a supportive environment by raising awareness regarding the benefits and importance of breastfeeding.

As we discuss the importance of breast feeding it is equally important for us to pivot and address some of the common myths surrounding breast feeding and what the truth is. Some people believe that breastfeeding is a reliable form of contraception. Though this is partially true, there is still high probability that a woman can get pregnant while she is breastfeeding. Therefore, it is essential to use a reliable form of contraception while breastfeeding. Lactating mothers should avoid estrogen containing oral contraceptive pills for at least 3-4 weeks post- partum. Another common myth and new mother concern is that small breasts do not produce sufficient milk. This is not true as the size of the breast does not determine the quantity of milk production. Milk production by the breasts is governed by a lot of factors which include adequate latching of the baby on the breasts, for sufficient time and on the frequency of breast feeding.

Once a mother is ready to breast feed and gears up for breast feeding, it is extremely important that the community supports this endeavor as the society plays a pivotal role in shaping attitudes and practices surrounding breastfeeding. Societal support helps in co-creating a conducive environment that extends beyond the immediate family. To establish societal encouragement and support, public health campaigns should be conducted to raise awareness on the benefits of breastfeeding and dispel any misconception regarding the same. Community outreach programs can provide a wonderful platform for lactating mothers to share their experiences and normalize the norms around breastfeeding by mitigating the stigma surrounding breastfeeding in public arenas. Inclusive strategies that encompass all strata of the population including healthcare workers, community leaders and social workers is necessary to establish a holistic support network for lactating mothers. And finally, as the mother transitions into this new phase of life, encouraging her to seek help and counselling regarding breastfeeding to establish a fulfilling and holistic experience is of paramount importance. Recognizing and championing the importance of breastfeeding portrays an investment in the foundation of a healthier and resilient global society.

7.

Lactation and the Solemnization of the Bond of Motherhood

Dr Aditya R. Nimbkar

M. S. (Obstetrics & Gynaecology)

As an obstetrician working in a medical college and a tertiary care hospital, this place is home to several meritorious residency programme students in our department of obstetrics and gynaecology. Known to be able to know the methods for managing the trickiest of obstetric emergencies, these students have a spark of brilliance to them, evidently visible. Be it a severely anaemic patient in labour, or an eclamptic, or a diabetic whose blood glucose levels are sky high, or even tough surgeries that can puzzle plenty, these residents can boast of being able to do most of it, if not all.

And yet, far often than not, with all their expertise in managing patients, there is a definite struggle when it comes to probably the least trained aspect of their patients, yet perhaps the most essential one for the patient herself and her newborn - lactation. A patient might have the smoothest of antenatal and intrapartum course, but what draws extreme anxiety for her, is the inability to feed her baby, immediately after birth.

Especially in primiparas, or simply put, women with their first birthing experience, this anxiety compounds further when the neonate develops hyperbilirubinemia, or jaundice due to lack of breastfeeding, as it lowers the enterohepatic cycling of the bile salts and pigments, and increases its absorption and eventual causation of jaundice that necessitates phototherapy on day 2 and 3 of delivery. And then commences a vicious circle of self-blame, thereby accentuating her own anxiety and stress, by the patient, in lieu of being incompetent towards her primary duty as a mother of being the sole provider of nutrition for her newborn. This results in further difficulty in lactation and can even land the female in postpartum depression!

And that is precisely where, a lactation consultant, or merely knowing the basics of breastfeeding by the one who is alongside the woman throughout the day, the obstetrics' resident, can rob this vicious cycle of the opportunity to reach calamitous proportions. And hence, it is pertinent that appropriate training of every doctor is undertaken, inculcating the skills in them to be able to encourage every female to lactate.

To begin with, the patient needs to be counselled regarding the magic potion, the unparalleled antidote to several neonatal and infantile illness, and perhaps the most underrated nectar of life, lies in the breastmilk that she secretes. The fat content of the breastmilk contains docosahexaenoic acid (DHA) and arachidonic acid, in amounts more significant than what formula feeds can provide, which help in the baby's neurological development. It is proven with evidence, that exclusive breastfeeding up to at least 6 months of age, can help have an average intelligence quotient (IQ), by 10 points more than those kids who were not breastfed at all. The breastmilk contains carbohydrates in the form of easily digestible lactose, and several proteins like alpha-lactalbumin, but in lower concentrations than cattle's milk, thereby not causing renal overload. Apart from micronutrients, like vitamins A, E and K, minerals like iron and zinc, presence of anti-infective agents like immunoglobulin A, oligosaccharides, lysozymes and lactoferrins, help in insuring the baby against several infective agents, and improving its gut immunity.

Once the patient has been explained these intricate nutritional advantages of breastmilk over cattle's milk or formula feeds, she can be assured of that fact that this unparalleled source of nutrition is supreme not just by the quality of it, but also the quantity that she can produce. The feeding is classically said to be 'demand feeding', which means that every time the baby seeks a feed, it must be readily given. And thankfully, pregnancy ensures that there's complete readiness of the breasts to augment this need that shall arise in the postpartum period by proliferation of the mammary glands. Proper positioning of the baby, is the most crucial step, in harnessing this wonderful gift of mother to her baby, by ensuring that the baby sucks milk from the breast, and not the nipple, in contrast to what many patients err at. A good attachment of the baby onto the breast consists of a fully open mouth of the baby, with the chin touching the breast, and the entirety of nipple and areola inside the mouth of the baby with the breast pulled out like funnel, and the baby's tongue with lashing movement on the inferior aspect of the breast up push it on his hard palate to express the breastmilk out from the lactiferous ducts.Pictorial presentation, by keeping readily visible pictures and charts in the maternity wards for public viewing, and demonstration of this process by a lactation consultant or the doctors, encourages mothers to feed, thereby making it a matter of pride for them to independently look after the nutritional demands of the baby.

A happy baby resides with a happy mother. Just like the umbilical cord connects the fetus intricately to the mother inside the womb, the baton is passed over to lactation to maintain that precious link when outside the womb. They say, *'nothing that this world provides, comes for free. And definitely not the good things'*. A mother though, chooses to be an aberration to this quote. The breastmilk, is the best thing that a mother can gift to her child, and this one come for free! Instead, the mother is the one who earns out of it, earning sheer satisfaction and joy, and a bond of motherhood, that stays miles ahead of any other bonds, unmatched.

So, in this annual breastfeeding week, let us pledge to educate ourselves about the significance of breastmilk and its feeding techniques and help the society conquer the ignominy of ignorance that exists around it.

8.

Promote Early Breastfeeding Along With Continued Breastfeeding

Ms Patricia Michael

Assistant Professor

Department of Nutrition

St. Francis College for Women, Hyderabad, Telangana India

Email: patricia.thomas0@gmail.com

Introduction

Breastfeeding is the basis of child, nourishment, survival, physical growth, and intellectual development. According to WHO (2009) breastfeeding exclusively during the initial six months of life, followed by a continuation of breastfeeding with adequate intake of foods up to two years or beyond.

Exclusive breastfeeding (EBF), during early childhood provides the much required essential nutrition for the infant, the initial six months is connected with a reduction in risk of neonatal sepsis, gastrointestinal infections , diarrhoea, respiratory infections , allergy, asthma, type I diabetes , obesity in later life , leukemia , and other non-communicable diseases (UNICEF/WHO, 2017).

The Indian scenario

The Health Ministry in India has given the topvalue to breast feeding intervention and is encouraging the States in realizing a nationwide programme named - 'MAA' (Mothers' Absolute Affection). This involves a thorough set of actions on promotion and support of breastfeeding at a community and facility level, through building an enabling environment.Reinforcing lactation support services at public health facilities through trained healthcare providers and awareness generation activities at community level.

Various regional studies across India have shown that several demographic factors such as physical health, education, maternal age, income, occupation, family size, Ante-Natal Checkup (ANC), and gender of the children are some of the important determinants of EBF.

The Government of India has taken up several projects, namely Pradhan Mantri SurakshitMatritva Abhiyan (PMSMA), Pradhan Mantri Matru Vandana Yojana (PMMVY), Maternity Leave Incentive Scheme, and Pan-India Maternity Benefits Program so that there is a development of maternal health during the gestational period, which is directly linked to newborn care, which includes breastfeeding. However, India has scored moderately in terms of Infant and Young Child Feeding (IYCF) policy, programs, and practice-according to the World Breastfeeding Trends Initiatives, 2018.

In the year 2016, India launched the Mothers' Absolute Affection (MAA) program, along with POSHAN Abhiyan to accelerate the ability and capacity of health workers concerning breastfeeding and IYCF practices.

The International viewpoint

The World Alliance for Breastfeeding Action (WABA) launched the Mother-Friendly Workplace Initiative (MFWI) as early as 1993 for worldwide response towards supporting working women's right to breast feed their infants.

Breastfeeding practices differ among the diverse countries of the world, according to UNICEF, 2018 about, 4% and 21% of infants from high-income countries and low-middle-income respectively, are never breastfed. However, globally, about 44% of children 0–5 months of age are breastfed exclusively, whereas it is slightly higher (57%) in Asian countries (UNICEF Data, 2019).

The young mothers and those who inhabitin ruralareas were found to be more informed with extended breastfecding practices. In a broader sense, there appears to a disparity between poor and rich communities in the practice of a continuation of breastfeeding up to 2 years of age all over the world. according to UNICEF 2018, only 57.7% of children in South Asia were reported to be breastfed among the richest quintile , whereas among the poor it was 81.3%.

World breastfeeding week 2023

The theme for World Breastfeeding Week this year 2023 is "Let's make breastfeeding and work, work!". The theme emphasises necessary measures to be taken bythe nation's policymakers, employers, and colleagues to strengthenthe practice of continued exclusive breastfeeding in working women to their babies.The theme also promotesan understanding regarding the value of optimal breastfeeding in infants and measures that will support working women.

Worldwide, thereare more than 50 crore working women are until now not having an access to vital maternity benefits, also several more who are not supported when they return to their workplaces.

As per WHO, every woman, wherever doing any job, ought to have the following:

- Paid maternity leave for at least 126 days (18 weeks) and ideally longer than six months.

- Paid lactation time off to nurse their kids.

- Provision of flexible return-to-work options

It is challenging for women working outside the home to combine breast feeding with their full-time employment. Breast feeding promotion and support in the workplace is important to encourage continued breast feeding among employed mothers. In order to successfully combine breast feeding with employment, the specific needs of the employed mothers should be contemplated in the workplace intervention programmes.

Understanding factors that influence EBF practices can contribute toward achieving the United Nations Sustainable Development Goal 3 (SGD3) - reducing neonatal mortality to at least as low as 12 neonatal deaths per 1000 live births by 2030.

9.

The Significance of Breastfeeding: A Comprehensive Comparison with Infant Formula Feeding

Anupreet Kaur Sobti

Ph.D. Research Scholar

Department of Foods and Nutrition, Government Home Science College, Chandigarh (Affiliated to Panjab University, Chandigarh), India

Introduction

The debate between breastfeeding and formula feeding has been ongoing for decades, with each method having its proponents and critics. While both options aim to nourish and sustain infants, breastfeeding stands out as a gold standard due to its numerous health benefits for both mothers and babies. This conceptual paper delves into the significance of breastfeeding, comparing it to infant formula feeding, and exploring the unique advantages that breast milk provides.

The biological significance of breast milk

Breast milk is a marvel of nature, specifically tailored to meet the nutritional needs of a newborn (Boquien, 2018). It contains a perfect blend of proteins, fats, carbohydrates, and micronutrients, all designed to support the rapid growth and development of a baby (Brockway et al., 2023). One of the most remarkable aspects of breast milk is its ability to adapt to the changing needs of the infant at different stages of development (Martin et al., 2016)

Breast milk is rich in antibodies and immune-boosting substances, providing infants with crucial protection against infections and diseases. The first milk produced, known as colostrum, is particularly potent in immune factors, aiding in the development of the baby's immune system. This natural defense mechanism is something that infant formula cannot replicate.

Nutritional composition: breast milk vs. Formula

While infant formula attempts to mimic the nutritional content of breast milk, it falls short in replicating the complexity and dynamic nature of breast milk. Breast milk contains live cells, hormones, enzymes, and other bioactive components (Ballard & Morrow, 2013) that contribute to the overall well-being of the baby. Formula, on the other hand, is a processed substitute that may lack some of these essential elements.

The fatty acids in breast milk, such as docosahexaenoic acid (DHA) and arachidonic acid

(ARA), are crucial for the development of the baby's brain and nervous system. Some formulas now include these components, but their synthetic nature may not be as easily absorbed by the baby's body.

The act of breastfeeding itself is more than just nutrition; it involves skin-to-skin contact, eye contact, and the release of bonding hormones like oxytocin (Modak et al., 2023). These emotional and physical aspects of breastfeeding contribute to the overall well-being of the child and strengthen the maternal-infant bond.

Health benefits for infants

Breastfeeding is associated with a myriad of health benefits for infants. Studies have shown that breastfed babies have a reduced risk of infections, allergies, and chronic diseases later in life. The antibodies present in breast milk help protect against respiratory infections, gastrointestinal issues, and ear infections.

Moreover, breastfeeding has been linked to a lower risk of sudden infant death syndrome (SIDS) (Hauck et al., 2011). The skin-to-skin contact during breastfeeding promotes the regulation of the baby's body temperature and helps establish a consistent sleep pattern.

Breastfeeding is also known to contribute to cognitive development. The fatty acids and other nutrients present in breast milk support optimal brain growth, potentially leading to higher IQ scores later in life (Belfort, 2017).

Health benefits for mothers

The benefits of breastfeeding extend beyond the infant to the mother. Breastfeeding helps in contracting the uterus after childbirth, reducing postpartum bleeding and aiding in a quicker recovery. It also helps mothers shed pregnancy weight more effectively (Makama et al., 2021).

Breastfeeding has long-term health advantages for mothers, reducing the risk of breast and ovarian cancers, as well as osteoporosis. The release of oxytocin during breastfeeding promotes a sense of well-being and reduces stress, contributing to the mother's emotional health (Matsunaga et al., 2020).

Economic and environmental considerations

Breastfeeding is not only beneficial for the health of infants and mothers but also has economic and environmental advantages (Binns et al., 2016). Breastfeeding is a cost-effective method of infant feeding, as breast milk is free and readily available. In contrast, formula feeding can be a considerable financial burden, with the cost of formula, bottles, and other feeding accessories.

Additionally, breastfeeding has a lower environmental impact compared to formula feeding. Formula production requires the use of resources, energy, and packaging, contributing to carbon footprints. Breastfeeding, being a natural process, is inherently eco-friendly.

Overcoming challenges and supporting breastfeeding

While the benefits of breastfeeding are evident, it's crucial to acknowledge that not every mother is able to breastfeed exclusively. Some face challenges such as latching difficulties, insufficient milk supply, or medical conditions that necessitate formula supplementation. In such cases, a supportive environment is essential to encourage and facilitate breastfeeding to the best extent possible.

Public policies that promote breastfeeding-friendly workplaces, extended maternity leave, and accessible lactation support can significantly contribute to the success of breastfeeding. Community support, education, and destigmatizing breastfeeding in public spaces are vital steps toward creating an environment where mothers feel empowered to breastfeed.

Conclusions

Breastfeeding stands as the optimal method of infant feeding, providing unparalleled health benefits for both infants and mothers. From the biological marvel of breast milk to the emotional and physical aspects of breastfeeding, the significance of this natural process cannot be overstated.

While infant formula serves as a valuable alternative in certain situations, it is essential to recognize the unique advantages of breast milk and work towards creating a supportive environment for breastfeeding mothers. By acknowledging and addressing the challenges that some mothers face, society can foster a culture that values and prioritizes breastfeeding, ultimately contributing to the health and well-being of future generations.

References

1. Ballard, O., & Morrow, A. L. (2013). Human milk composition. *Pediatric Clinics of North America*, *60*(1), 49–74. https://doi.org/10.1016/j.pcl.2012.10.002

2. Belfort, M. B. (2017). The science of breastfeeding and brain development. *Breastfeeding Medicine*, *12*(8), 459–461. https://doi.org/10.1089/bfm.2017.0122

3. Binns, C., Lee, M. K., & Low, W. Y. (2016). The Long-Term Public Health Benefits of Breastfeeding. *Asia Pacific Journal of Public Health*, *28*(1), 7–14. https://doi.org/10.1177/1010539515624964

4. Boquien, C. (2018). Human milk: an ideal food for nutrition of preterm newborn. *Frontiers in Pediatrics*, 6. https://doi.org/10.3389/fped.2018.00295

5. Brockway, M., Daniel, A. I., Reyes, S. M., Granger, M., McDermid, J. M., Chan, D., Refvik, R., Sidhu, K. K., Musse, S., Patel, P. P., Monnin, C., Lotoski, L., Geddes, D. T., Jehan, F., Kolsteren, P., Allen, L. H., Hampel, D., Eriksen, K. G., Rodriguez, N., & Azad, M. B. (2023). Human milk macronutrients and child growth and body composition in the first 2 years: a systematic review. *Advances in Nutrition,*

100149. https://doi.org/10.1016/j.advnut.2023.100149

6. Hauck, F. R., Thompson, J. M. D., Tanabe, K. O., Moon, R. Y., & Vennemann, M. (2011). Breastfeeding and reduced risk of sudden infant death Syndrome: A Meta-analysis. *Pediatrics, 128*(1), 103–110. https://doi.org/10.1542/peds.2010-3000

7. Makama, M., Skouteris, H., Moran, L. J., & Lim, S. (2021). Reducing Postpartum Weight Retention: A review of the implementation challenges of postpartum lifestyle interventions. *Journal of Clinical Medicine, 10*(9), 1891. https://doi.org/10.3390/jcm10091891

8. Martin, C. R., Ling, P., & Blackburn, G. L. (2016). Review of infant feeding: Key features of breast milk and infant formula. *Nutrients, 8*(5), 279. https://doi.org/10.3390/nu8050279

9. Matsunaga, M., Kikusui, T., Mogi, K., Nagasawa, M., Ooyama, R., &Myowa, M. (2020). Breastfeeding dynamically changes endogenous oxytocin levels and emotion recognition in mothers. *Biology Letters, 16*(6), 20200139. https://doi.org/10.1098/rsbl.2020.0139

10. Modak, A., Ronghe, V., &Gomase, K. (2023). The Psychological Benefits of Breastfeeding: Fostering Maternal Well-Being and Child Development. *Cureus.* https://doi.org/10.7759/cureus.46730

10.
Nurturing Breastfeeding Support in the Indian Context: A Conceptual Framework

Dr. Anjali Juyal

Guest Faculty

Department of Resource Management and Consumer Science

CCAS, MPUAT, Udaipur

Email: anjalijuyal1994@gmail.com

Abstract

In the culturally rich and diverse landscape of India, the journey of motherhood is intertwined with various traditions and challenges. One crucial aspect of this journey is breastfeeding, which not only nurtures the infant but also forms a profound connection between mother and child. However, for many mothers in India, the path of breastfeeding is laden with obstacles. This paper explores the importance of breastfeeding support emphasizing the need for accessible and close support systems in the culturally diverse and dynamic context of India. Recognizing the unique challenges faced by mothers in this setting, the paper introduces a comprehensive conceptual framework designed to foster and enhance breastfeeding support systems. Drawing on insights from healthcare professionals, communities, employers, and policymakers, this framework envisions a collaborative and holistic approach that transcends traditional boundaries.

Introduction

Commencing breastfeeding within the initial hour of birth and providing the infant with colostrum, a rich and nutritious secretion, are crucial steps in establishing a robust foundation for a healthy life during infancy and beyond. According to recommendations from the World Health Organization (WHO) and UNICEF, exclusive breastfeeding, meaning no additional food or drink, not even water, should be practiced for the first 6 months. The breastfeeding regimen should be based on the infant's demand, and the use of bottles, teats, or pacifiers should be avoided. Subsequently, from 6 months onwards, age-appropriate complementary foods should be introduced while continuing breastfeeding until the child reaches 2 years or beyond.

Providing adequate nutrition, care, protection, love, and affection is fundamental for the child's proper growth and development. In India, breastfeeding mothers encounter a spectrum of challenges, ranging from cultural expectations to lack of awareness about best practices. Understanding the emotional and physical aspects of breastfeeding is crucial for providing tailored support. Many mothers face uncertainties and anxieties, making the role of support systems even more critical in their breastfeeding journey.

Breastfeeding, a natural and fundamental aspect of motherhood, is interwoven with a tapestry of cultural, societal, and individual nuances in the diverse landscape of India. To establish a robust conceptual framework for nurturing breastfeeding support, it is imperative to delve deeply into the multifaceted challenges confronted by breastfeeding mothers, encompassing both the emotional and physical dimensions of their journey.

1. Emotional challenges

Indian cultural norms significantly impact a mother's decision and ability to breastfeed, creating emotional challenges as mothers navigate conflicting expectations and perceptions imposed by societal pressures.Breastfeeding's emotional toll extends to a mother's mental well-being, influencing confidence and commitment. Anxiety, self-doubt, and postpartum emotional fluctuations are crucial emotional nuances requiring understanding for effective support.Emotional experiences are shaped by interpersonal relationships, especially support from family members. Lack of understanding or encouragement, particularly from spouses and extended family, can contribute to emotional stress, hindering the breastfeeding experience.

2. Physical challenges

Breastfeeding, while natural, presents physiological challenges like latch difficulties, engorgement, and nipple pain, potentially deterring mothers. Recognizing and addressing these physical barriers are crucial for establishing an effective support foundation.The mother's physical well-being profoundly impacts breastfeeding success. Maternal health factors, including postpartum recovery, nutritional status, and pre-existing health conditions, directly influence breastfeeding ability. A comprehensive understanding of these factors is vital for tailored support.Critical to breastfeeding success is the health of the infant. Mothers may face challenges if infants experience difficulties in latching, feeding, or have specific health issues. Addressing these concerns necessitates a holistic approach, considering both the mother and infant's well-being.

Strategies for nurturing breastfeeding

Developing effective policies for breastfeeding involves creating a supportive environment that encourages and facilitates breastfeeding for mothers. Here are key policy areas that can contribute to fostering breastfeeding support:

1. Workplace policies

Extending maternity leave ensures that mothers have sufficient time to initiate breastfeeding routines and recover from childbirth. Allowing flexible work hours or part-time schedules accommodates breastfeeding mothers by providing flexibility around their infants' feeding schedules. The mandate to create lactation rooms with comfortable seating, privacy, and electrical outlets for breast pumps facilitates a conducive space for mothers to express milk while at work. Additionally, providing dedicated breastfeeding breaks during working hours acknowledges the importance of regular breastfeeding or expressing sessions for nursing mothers. These policies collectively contribute to creating a workplace that prioritizes the well-being of breastfeeding mothers, supporting their ability to maintain a breastfeeding relationship with their infants while fulfilling professional responsibilities.

2. Public spaces

Promoting breastfeeding-friendly spaces in public areas is crucial for supporting nursing mothers. Encouraging businesses, malls, and public places to designate specific areas with comfortable seating and privacy fosters an environment where mothers can comfortably breastfeed. Simultaneously, public awareness campaigns play a pivotal role in educating the community about the importance of creating a supportive atmosphere for breastfeeding in public spaces. These initiatives collectively contribute to normalizing breastfeeding, empowering mothers to feed their infants comfortably and confidently in various public settings.

3. Healthcare settings

Promoting breastfeeding-friendly spaces in public areas is crucial for supporting nursing mothers. Encouraging businesses, malls, and public places to designate specific areas with comfortable seating and privacy fosters an environment where mothers can comfortably breastfeed. Simultaneously, public awareness campaigns play a pivotal role in educating the community about the importance of creating a supportive atmosphere for breastfeeding in public spaces. These initiatives collectively contribute to normalizing breastfeeding, empowering mothers to feed their infants comfortably and confidently in various public settings.

4. Community initiatives

Community initiatives play a pivotal role in bolstering breastfeeding support. Establishing breastfeeding support groups within communities fosters a network of assistance and shared experiences, providing mothers with valuable guidance. Simultaneously, community-based educational programs are essential for informing families about the numerous benefits of breastfeeding and dispelling common misconceptions. By facilitating the formation of support groups and implementing educational initiatives at the community level, a supportive environment is created, promoting breastfeeding as a norm and empowering families with the knowledge and resources necessary for a positive breastfeeding experience.

5. Employer support

Encouraging employer support is pivotal for fostering a breastfeeding-friendly workplace. Offering incentives or recognition for companies that actively support breastfeeding employees, including policies like flexible working arrangements and dedicated lactation facilities, serves as a positive reinforcement.

Additionally, conducting training programs for managers and human resources personnel is essential. These programs equip them with the knowledge and skills needed to provide meaningful support to breastfeeding employees, contributing to the creation of a workplace culture that not only accommodates but actively promotes the well-being of nursing mothers, thereby enhancing the overall work environment.

6. Educational institutions

Creating a supportive environment for student mothers is crucial, and establishing policies that address their unique needs is a significant step. By implementing provisions such as dedicated lactation rooms and flexible class schedules, educational institutions can ensure that student mothers have the necessary facilities and flexibility to balance their academic commitments with breastfeeding responsibilities. These policies acknowledge the importance of supporting student mothers in continuing their education while also attending to the needs of their infants. By fostering an inclusive educational environment, institutions contribute to the overall well-being and success of student mothers pursuing their academic goals.

7. Research and monitoring

Prioritizing research and monitoring in breastfeeding initiatives is essential for evidence-based policy development. Supporting research initiatives to collect data on breastfeeding rates, challenges, and success factors enables policymakers to make informed decisions and adjustments. Additionally, implementing robust monitoring and evaluation mechanisms ensures ongoing assessment of the effectiveness of existing breastfeeding policies. Regular evaluations identify areas for improvement, allowing for dynamic adjustments to policies and programs. By emphasizing data collection and evaluation, stakeholders can continuously refine strategies, ultimately fostering a more supportive and adaptive framework for breastfeeding initiatives.

8. Legal protections

Ensuring legal protections is paramount for breastfeeding mothers. Strengthening anti-discrimination laws safeguards nursing mothers from discrimination in various settings, including workplaces, public spaces, and educational institutions. These legal measures send a clear message that breastfeeding is a protected right, and individuals should not face discrimination for exercising it.

Similarly, establishing explicit laws ensuring the right to breastfeed in public without harassment or discrimination further normalizes breastfeeding practices, fostering an inclusive and supportive environment. By fortifying legal protections, policymakers contribute to creating a society where breastfeeding mothers can confidently and comfortably fulfill their maternal responsibilities without fear of prejudice or discrimination.

9. Insurance coverage

Expanding insurance coverage to include lactation consultant services is a pivotal step in promoting comprehensive maternal and infant health. By incorporating coverage for lactation consultants under health insurance plans, mothers gain access to professional guidance crucial for successful breastfeeding. This initiative acknowledges the significance of specialized support during the breastfeeding journey, enhancing accessibility for women seeking expert assistance. The inclusion of such services in insurance coverage not only prioritizes maternal and infant well-being but also contributes to normalizing and encouraging breastfeeding practices by ensuring that mothers have the necessary resources for a positive breastfeeding experience.

These policies, when implemented and enforced effectively, can contribute to creating a supportive and encouraging environment for breastfeeding mothers across various sectors of society.

Harnessing digital connectivity: empowering breastfeeding support in the digital era

In an age defined by digital connectivity, the conceptual framework seamlessly incorporates online resources as a pivotal component, recognizing their transformative potential. Virtual lactation consultations emerge as dynamic channels, transcending physical limitations and bringing expert guidance directly to breastfeeding mothers, irrespective of their geographical locations. Interactive platforms and forums play a crucial role in building a virtual community where mothers can share insights, seek advice, and find solidarity in their breastfeeding experiences.

By breaking down traditional barriers, this integration ensures that mothers across the expanse of India have accessible and immediate support at their fingertips. The framework thus leverages the power of technology to create a digital ecosystem that not only disseminates knowledge but also fosters a sense of connectivity and support, transcending the constraints of physical distance and enriching the breastfeeding experience for mothers in the digital age.

Government initiatives: catalyzing nationwide breastfeeding support

Within the conceptual framework, a crucial aspect involves integrating government initiatives to propel comprehensive breastfeeding support across the nation. This section envisions a multifaceted approach, advocating for national campaigns, funding programs, and the seamless integration of breastfeeding education into broader public health initiatives. Recognizing the pivotal role of government involvement, this component becomes a linchpin for amplifying the impact of breastfeeding support on a nationwide scale.

1. National campaigns

Spearheading the strategy, national campaigns aim to raise awareness about breastfeeding's importance, utilizing various mediums to disseminate evidence-based information and foster a cultural shift in support. By leveraging their extensive reach, the framework strives for a widespread understanding of breastfeeding's benefits across diverse regions.

2. Funding programs

Recognizing financial considerations, the framework advocates dedicated funding programs to allocate resources for lactation support services, community workshops, and healthcare professional training. Securing financial backing aims to fortify infrastructure for effective breastfeeding support mechanisms in urban and rural settings.

3. Integration into public health initiatives

This strategic synergy integrates breastfeeding education seamlessly into broader public health initiatives. By incorporating guidance into routine maternal and child health programs, the framework addresses the well-being of mothers and infants, fostering a culture of sustained maternal and infant health as an intrinsic part of overall healthcare.

4. Policy advocacy

Beyond specific programs, the framework emphasizes policy advocacy, engaging policymakers to shape and strengthen legislative frameworks supporting breastfeeding-friendly environments. This involves advocating for workplace policies, public spaces conducive to breastfeeding, and legal frameworks protecting the rights of breastfeeding mothers.

Government initiatives and policies promoting breastfeeding in India

India has implemented several policies and initiatives to promote and support breastfeeding. It's important to note that government policies can evolve, and there may be new developments or changes after my last update. Here are some key initiatives and policies related to breastfeeding in India:

1. National guidelines on infant and young child feeding

The Ministry of Women and Child Development in India has issued National Guidelines on Infant and Young Child Feeding. These guidelines provide recommendations and strategies for promoting optimal feeding practices, including breastfeeding.

2. Mother's absolute affection (MAA) program

The Mother's Absolute Affection (MAA) program was launched by the Ministry of Health and Family Welfare. It aims to promote and support breastfeeding through various interventions, including community awareness campaigns, training healthcare providers, and encouraging maternity hospitals to adopt breastfeeding-friendly practices.

3. Poshan abhiyaan (National nutrition mission)

The Poshan Abhiyaan, or National Nutrition Mission, includes breastfeeding promotion as a key component. It focuses on improving maternal and child nutrition, emphasizing the importance of exclusive breastfeeding during the first six months of life.

4. Baby-friendly hospital initiative (BFHI)

India has been working on implementing the BFHI in maternity hospitals to ensure that healthcare facilities support breastfeeding initiation and continuation. BFHI practices promote skin-to-skin contact, rooming-in, and early initiation of breastfeeding.

5. Maternity benefit (amendment) act

The Maternity Benefit (Amendment) Act in India has provisions for maternity leave, which is crucial for supporting breastfeeding mothers. It extends the duration of maternity leave and ensures that women have the time and support needed to breastfeed their infants.

6. National health mission (NHM)

The National Health Mission in India has been involved in various maternal and child health programs, which include components related to promoting breastfeeding awareness and support.

These policies and programs reflect the Indian government's commitment to improving maternal and child health outcomes by supporting breastfeeding. For the most current and detailed information, it is recommended to check official government health websites, publications, or contact relevant government authorities in the Ministry of Health and Family Welfare and the Ministry of Women and Child Development.

Challenges and solutions

Tailoring solutions to address the distinctive challenges faced in the Indian context is imperative for fostering successful breastfeeding support. This component of the conceptual framework underscores the need for a collaborative and inclusive approach that engages diverse stakeholders. Recognizing the multifaceted nature of challenges, the framework advocates for the active involvement of healthcare professionals, employers, community leaders, and other relevant entities. Educational campaigns take center stage, disseminating targeted information and promoting awareness about breastfeeding best practices. Workplace policies are envisaged to create supportive environments that accommodate the unique needs of nursing mothers. Simultaneously, community-based initiatives are integrated to establish a localized network of support, acknowledging the communal nature of Indian society. By fostering collaboration among these stakeholders, the framework aims to create a unified and adaptive strategy, ensuring that the solutions developed are not only effective but also culturally sensitive, addressing the specific challenges encountered by mothers navigating the intricate landscape of breastfeeding in India.

Conclusions

In the culturally rich and diverse landscape of India, breastfeeding is a crucial aspect of the intricate journey of motherhood. This paper delves into the challenges faced by Indian mothers in their breastfeeding journey and emphasizes the need for accessible and close support systems. A comprehensive conceptual framework is introduced, advocating for collaboration and tailored solutions from diverse stakeholders, including healthcare professionals, communities, employers, and policymakers. This framework envisions a holistic approach that transcends traditional boundaries, recognizing the unique challenges faced by mothers in the dynamic Indian context. It explores the emotional and physical challenges of breastfeeding, underlining the significance of support systems. It discusses the components of healthcare professionals' roles, community-based initiatives, digital connectivity, and government involvement, all crucial elements within the framework. The framework seeks to create an environment where breastfeeding is not only normalized but ingrained into the fabric of public health, contributing to the overall well-being of mothers and infants across diverse regions of the country.

References

1. Child Health Division Ministry of Health and Family Welfare Government of India. 2017. National Guidelines on Lactation Management Centres in Public Health Facilities. Retrieved from on https://nhm.gov.in/images/pdf/programmes/IYCF/National_Guidelines_Lactation_Management_Centres.pdf on 12/01/2024.

2. World Health Organization. 2020. Baby-friendly Hospital Initiative training course for maternity staff: customisation Guide. Retrieved from https://www.who.int/publications/i/item/9789240008915 on 12/01/2024

3. Escamilla, R. P., Tomori, C., Cordero, S. H., Baker,P., Barros, A. J. D., Bégin,F., Chapman,D.J., Strawn, L. M. G., McCoy,D., Menon,P., Neves, P.A.R., Piwoz,E., Rollins,N., Victora, C. G. and Richter, L. 2023. Breastfeeding: crucially important, but increasingly challenged in a market-driven world. *The lancet.***401**(10375):472-485.

4. Samaniego, J. A. R., Maramag, C.C., Castro, M. C., Zambrano, P., Nguyen, T.T., Sanguyo, J. D., Cashin, D. J. and Mathisen, R. and Weissman, A. 2022. Implementation and Effectiveness of Policies Adopted to Enable Breastfeeding in the Philippines Are Limited by Structural and Individual Barriers. *International Journal of Environmental Research and Public Health.* **19**(17): 10938.

5. National Health Mission. 2016. Programme for Promotion of Breastfeeding: Operational Guidelines. Retrieved from https://nhm.gov.in/MAA/Operational_Guidelines.pdf on 17/01/2024.

6. UNICEF. 2018. Protecting, promoting and supporting Breastfeeding in facilities providing maternity and newborn services: the revised BABY-FRIENDLY HOSPITAL INITIATIVE. Retrieved from https://www.unicef.org/media/95191/file/Baby-friendly-hospital-initiative-implementation-guidance-2018.pdf on 20/01/2024.

7. Passi, S.J. and Jain, A. Why do we need to promote breastfeeding? Retrieved from https://pib.gov.in/newsite/printrelease.aspx?relid=169387 on 24/01/2024.

8. Krol, K.M and Grossmann, T. 2018. Psychological effects of breastfeeding on children and mothers. *BundesgesundheitsblattGesundheitsforschungGesundheitsschutz (Federal Health Bulletin - Health Research - Health Protection).* 61(8): 977–985.

9. Rivi, V., Petrilli,G. and Blom, M.C.J. 2020.Mind the Mother When Considering Breastfeeding. *Frontiers Global Womens Health*. Retrieved from https://www.frontiersin.org/articles/10.3389/fgwh.2020.0000 3/full on 26/01/2024.

11.

The Nurturing Bond: A Mother's Journey Through Breastfeeding

Dr. Uzma Mustaq

Researcher

Institute of Home science, University of Kashmir Hazratbal Srinagar, Jammu and Kashmir, India

Email: Uzmanaqash19@gmail.com

Keywords: Breastfeeding, Experiences, First year, Mothers, Preterm infant

Breastfeeding is among the newborn's first experiences supporting optimal short- and long –term-health. **(Victora et al., 2016)** Breastfeeding journey of mothers during the first year after a pretermbirth has not been well studied.it was described as a way to rest and calm down as well as a period of relaxation for both the mother and infant. In this study, exclusive breastfeeding was defined as feeding with breast milk only regardless of feeding method, but could include medications, fortification and vitamins. Partial breastfeeding was defined as feeding with breast milk in combination with formula and /or solid food.

Human experience is complex and cannot be understood by analyzing parts or measuring aspects of breastfeeding, as we are also affected by social context. It is important to assess each mother's experience of breastfeeding their preterm infant because each individual mother has the most knowledge about her own experience. Illuminating breastfeeding may help health professionals to provide caring and supportive relationships through learning about the mothers' individual experiences. Thus, the aim of this study was to describe mothers' experiences of breastfeeding their preterm infants from birth up until 12 months after birth. **(Lina Palmér et al., 2019)**

Navigating smoothly

Navigating smoothly through one's breastfeeding journey means that breastfeeding was experienced in a positive way without any major problems or difficulties. breastfeeding was a way to become close withthe infant and thus strengthen the relationship between the mother and infant. The mothers experienced a feeling of togetherness with their infants. They described this feeling of togetherness as a mutual interaction and an intimate relationship with the infant. Such mutuality and intimacy was reported to provide a unique closeness and strong bond with the infant.The mothers also described breastfeeding as a gift to the infant. Breastfeeding gave the mothers a lovely feeling, and it was satisfying to provide the infant with nutrition and protection, which was perceived as being the best possible start. It was described as "awesome" and "beautiful" when the infant became satisfied by being breastfed.

Navigating with a struggle

Navigating with a struggle means that the breastfeeding journey is experienced more or less as a bodily performance instead of a smooth relationship with the infant. The most prominent problem or difficulty faced by the mothers was that the infants' prematurity complicated breastfeeding. The mothers reported that their infants could not or did not want to breastfeed. The infants could have a weak suck or did not suck. The interaction and relationship between the mother and infant were, or could be, complicated. Sometimes, the mother wanted to breastfeed but the infant did not. Struggling with breastfeeding may also be associated with having too much milk and thus being confronted with extreme bodily changes in the breasts. Such bodily changes in the breast may in some cases be experienced as very trying and, in some cases, these changes of the breast can be perceived as disgusting.

Breastfeeding was sometimes seen as an exhausting situation that caused the mothers to experience stress. Furthermore, feelings of failure, of being solely responsible, being insufficient or incapable were also expressed. These feelings sometimes led to disappointment and frustration that breastfeeding did not work out as expected. Breastfeeding was reported by some mothers to be mentally tough and unpredictable; moreover, the need to always be close to the infant and the inability to leave was tiring for some mothers.

Furthermore, when comparing other research about mothers' experiences of breastfeeding their preterm infants, it seems that breastfeeding mothers of preterm infants in different Western countries experience certain similarities. A recurrent issue in the studies, including ours, was that the infant's prematurity complicated breastfeeding. This issue could be addressed in neonatal care to identify care routines that support the preterm infant's development as well as to educate parents about preterm infant feeding development and how to support the infant during breastfeeding. In some other countries, it is more common to feed infants expressed breast milk in a bottle for various reasons, including care routines, society norms and/or personal reasons.

Conclusions

Mothers journey breastfeeding their preterm infants in different ways, and each mother found her own way in breastfeeding. An awareness of the diversity of breastfeeding experiences may help provide better professional caring and supporting relationships. The whole care chain for preterm infants and their mothers (e.g., maternity, neonatal and child health care) needs to have a caring approach and holistically meet the uniqueness in every mother's breastfeeding situation.

References

1. C.G victora, r. bahl, A.J,Barros, G.V Franca,S. Horton,J. Krasevec,S. Murch,M.J. Sankar, N.walker,N.C.Rollins. (2016) breastfeeding in the 2ist century: epidemiology, mechanisms, and lifelong effect. Pp.475-490
2. Ericson J, Palmer L. (2019) Mothers of preterm infants' experiences of breastfeeding support in

the first 12 months after birth: a qualitative study. Birth.46, pp.129–36

3. Palmer L, Carlsson G, Mollberg M, Nystrom M. (2012) Severe breastfeeding difficulties: existential lostness as a mother-women's lived experiences of initiating breastfeeding under severe difficulties. Int J Qual Stud Health Well-being. 27, pp.108-46

12
Breastfeeding Support: Close to Mothers

Pooja R Singhania

PhD (Food Science & Nutrition)

Certified Infant & Young Child Feeding Counseling Specialist by BPNI

Certified MIYCN expert by IIT Mumbai

Founder, Nourish 1000 Days

Email: nourish1000days@gmail.com

Have you heard of the famous proverb "It takes a village to raise a child" . This proverb indicates how valuable the support and guidance of the community is to the family that is raising a child. Because no matter how much knowledge we have tried to gather from resources such as books, magazines, media, etc eventually when the baby is born- every mother needs support

In my own experience, despite being a PhD in Food Science & Nutrition and knowing that breastfeeding is the best form of nutrition for a baby, I was struggling with breastfeeding. And when I was almost about to give up on breastfeeding and give in to the pressure to use breastmilk substitutes (e.g. formula milk), I found the much needed SUPPORT. Yes, a friend who is a Maternal and Child Nutrition expert finally guided me on the right technique of breastfeeding and I could sustain it. Soon after that one conversation with her, I was convinced that there is no way other than breastfeeding. Just keep feeding, feeding, and feeding!

Ironically, this same friend of mine, when she delivered her first baby, needed my support and guidance. At the Hospital itself she was misguided that her newborn daughter needed top feed (formula milk) otherwise she may not survive. My friend was in a vulnerable state post delivery but she reached out for support to the Breastfeeding experts and took a stance that went against the advice of Doctors at the Hospital. She continued to provide her own breast milk only and ensured that the baby was by her side at all times so that no one could give her breast milk substitute.

These experiences were enough to help me understand the importance of a strong SUPPORT system for a new mother and baby. That time the decision was made to start Free Mother Support groups!

Mother support groups are platforms (online and sometimes offline) wherein mothers can join for free and post their questions. They can have simple doubts cleared and queries addressed. Questions which may seem too simple or trivial, but are actually of great concern to the mother can be asked freely.

E.g. My breastfed baby has not passed motion for the past 3 days. What can I do?

My baby seems to be putting hands into her mouth too often, does it mean she is hungry?

My baby is feeding every hour, is my milk supply not enough for her?

Advantages of mother support groups

1. Time saving & fast

For such small questions, mothers are not able to contact their Gynecologists or Pediatricians. These professionals may not be available or easily approachable. Visiting the Doctor for such doubts at their clinic may also not be practical for a new mother. Hence, the online support platforms are extremely useful.Even in the middle of the night, a mother might find help from a fellow mother and feel a bit relaxed.

2. Feeling of safety

When mothers ask questions within such communities, they are assured that there is no misuse of information. They also feel safe to share images of babies freely. Mothers might have to share personal information also and they feel it is safe to share with fellow mothers

3. Non-judgmental

In mother support groups, mothers do not judge each other. One mother understands the challenges of the other, and gives her a practical solution. There is empathy amongst fellow mothers so before telling her that what she is doing is wrong or foolish, they try to understand why she has taken such a decision

4. Confidence

While mothers ask their trivial questions on the support groups, they realize that they are not the only ones facing that particular problem. The same doubts and concerns are there in the mind of fellow mothers also. Most babies of the same age exhibit similar behaviors. E.g. At 6 weeks, babies start appearing to be fussy and feed at frequent intervals. Mothers get very tired and often start doubting whether their milk supply is sufficient for their baby or not. At such times, when fellow mothers of same age babies share that they are experiencing the same thing, mothers feel assured. They realize that the problem is not with them, it is a phase that baby is going through.

We always use this saying in our groups **"THIS TOO SHALL PASS"**.

Mothers understand that what is happening is normal and just a phase. It makes them relaxed and feel more confident.

Possible drawbacks of mother support groups

1. Authentic experts

Sometimes, commercial sites which sell baby products start WhatsApp support groups with the intention to sell their products. It could be pumps, bottles, formula milk, diapers, etc. Such support groups might be managed by unqualified people who may have limited knowledge of Infant & Young Child Feeding Practices. Such support groups must be avoided . Ensure that you are receiving information from well qualified experts only.

A word of caution here is that even Gynaecologist and Pediatricians gain very limited information about breastfeeding through their medical curriculum. Hence, they are not very well equipped to handle breastfeeding challenges. Look for experts who have undergone training such as the

- Infant & Young Child feeding counseling specialist curse by BPNI, India

- Maternal Infant & Young CHild Nutrition experts by IIT Mumbai

- Certified Lactation Professionals /Advanced Certified Lactation professionals by BegnEd India

- International board certified Lactation consultants by WABA

2. Negative comments

The administrators of the support groups need to be constantly vigilant about keeping the vibes of the group positive and productive. Unnecessary comments, marketing and gossip must be kept under check. There needs to be strict Rules and Regulation of the group which must be followed by all. Any comments that makes another lose her confidence or feel inadequate must be avoided.

List of some authentic support groups on various media platforms

<u>Offline-</u>

Mother Support Group by BPNI , Maharashtra

<u>**Online-**</u>

Facebook

Breastfeeding support for Indian mothers

Breastfeeding & Pumping Support:India

Live Love Babywear

WhatsApp support groups

Lactation Matters

Nourish 1000 Days

Helpline

Maa Aur Shishu Poshan

As a New Mother we get a lot of advice. It is time to get more support. You seek support and it will surely come to you. Do not hesitate to have the smallest of queries resolved. Remember, you will do what is best for your child but with the right knowledge, you will be saved from regrets later on.

13.

Need of Homoeopathic Remedies for Lactating Mothers

Dr. Chetna Rochani

MD (Hom), PG-FHPC, N.D.D.Y.

Associate Professor & HOD, Department of Pathology

P P Savani University, Kosamba, Surat.

Email: drchetnarochani18@gmail.com

Abstract

Breastfeeding is a significant event in woman's life. Every woman expects that her pregnancy, delivery as well lactation period should be smooth and uneventful, where mother as well baby both can enjoy their existence and their health at the peak.If we talk about lactation then various factors play significant role in breast feeding, like general condition of mother, psychological state of mother, quantity of milk, quality of milk, condition of breast and nipples as well baby's general condition etc. Breast milk not only provides a baby with ideal nutrition and immunity but also supports growth, development as well bonding between mother and child. Must not forget that, mother's psychological state directly affects her child during lactation period. In this article, I have highlighted common problems during lactation and its prompt solution with Homeopathic remedies.

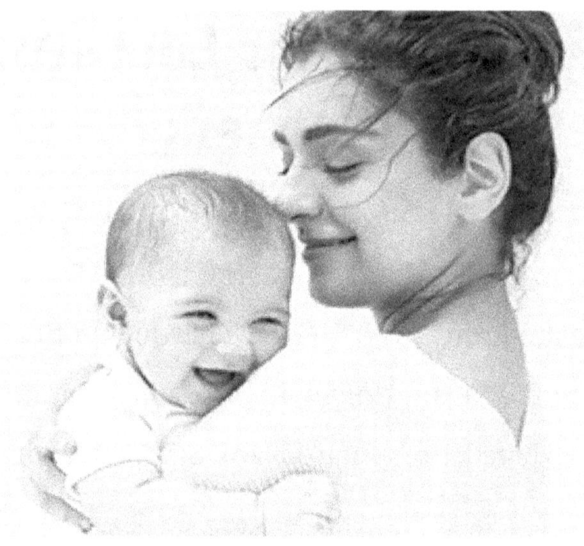

Key words: Lactation, Breastfeeding, Deficient Milk, Mastitis, Homoeopathy.

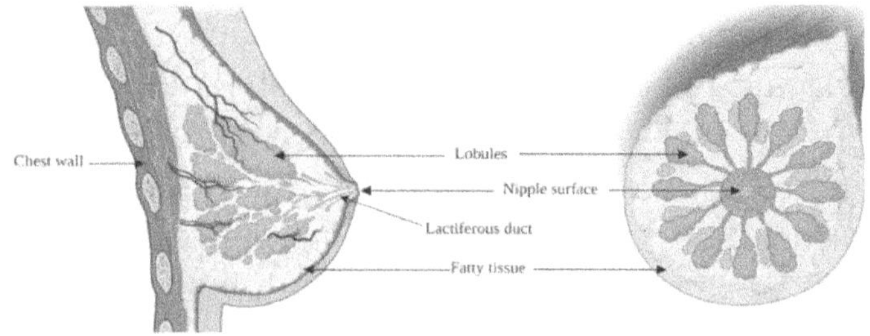

Introduction

The breast is a modified skin appendage which is functional in the females during lactation.Its major function is to provide for the nutritional support and survival of the infant. Microanatomy of the breast

76

reveals 2 types of tissue components: Epithelial and Stromal. Inflammation of the breast is called mastitis. Important types of mastitis are acute mastitis, breast abscess, chronic mastitis, traumatic fat necrosis and galactocele. Often, women stop because these common problems interfere with their ability to breastfeed. Homoeopathic medicines help to overcome these obstacles.

Homoeopathic remedies for lactating mothers

Here are few Homoeopathic medicines that can be utilised with prompt effect and best results.

1. Alfalfa

Increases quality and quantity of milk in nursing mothers. If a baby has failure to thrive, Alfalfa favourably influences nutrition, evidenced in "toning up" the appetite and digestion resulting in greatly improved mental and physical vigor, with gain in weight. Acts as a fat producer, corrects tissue waste.

2. Belladonna

MASTITIS, pain, throbbing, redness, streaks radiate from nipple. Breasts feel heavy, hard and red. Tumors of breast, pain worse lying down.

3. Borax veneta

Apthae in the mouth, on the tongue, inside of cheeks, easily bleeding when touched, prevents child from nursing, with hot mouth. Tremendous fear of downward motion. Also in woman, breasts are painful during nursing, aching after nursing. When nursing, pain in opposite breast.

4. Bryonia Alba

BREASTS HOT AND PAINFUL, HARD (Mastitis). Abscess of mammae. Milk fever.

5. Conium Maculatum

Mammae lax and shrunken, hard, painful to touch, mastitis, stiches in the mammae and nipples on taking deep breathing or walking. Wants to press the breast hard with the hand.

6. Silica

Fistulous ulcers of breast. Discharge of blood from vagina every time child is nursed. Hard lumps in breast.

7. Phytolacca

HEAVY, STONY, HARD SWOLLEN OR TENDER MAMMAE; paining during suckling; spreading all over the body. Hard nodes in breast; with enlarged axillary glands. Nipples; cracked, very sensitive; inverted. Galactorrhoea. Bloody, watery discharge from mammae. Affection of old cicatrices in mammae.

8. Urtica urens

Diminished secretion of milk; after parturition. Swelling of the breast; with stinging, burning pains. Arrests the flow of milk after weaning.

References

1. Mohan Harsh, Text Book of Pathology, Edition 7th, Jaypee Brothers Medical Publishers (P) Ltd, p. 745
2. Robbins & Cortan, Pathologic Basis of disease, Elsevier, 2021, p. 1037
3. *Boericke William, New manual of homoeopathic materia Medica & Repertory, B Jain Publishers Pvt Ltd. 2001, p.27, p.112, p.132, p. 225, p.573*
4. Phatak S.R., Materia Medica of Homeopathic Medicines, IBPP, 2011, p.108, p.214, p 606, p.469, p.392
5. Allen H.C, Allen's Keynotes and Characteristics with withNosodes, B. Jain Publishers Pvt. Ltd, 2002, P. 63

14.

Breastfeeding in Special Circumstances: Nurturing Health against All Odds

Dr. Ritu Pradhan

Head and Associate Professor

Department of Foods and Nutrition, Government Home Science College, Chandigarh (Affiliated to Panjab University, Chandigarh), India

Introduction

Breastfeeding is a cornerstone of infant health, providing unparalleled nutrition and immunity that contribute to a child's growth and well-being. In special circumstances, such as premature births, maternal health issues, or infants with medical conditions, breastfeeding takes on an even more significant role. This conceptual paper explores the challenges and importance of breastfeeding in special circumstances, shedding light on how this natural process can be a lifeline for infants facing unique health challenges.

Breastfeeding premature infants

Premature birth brings its own set of challenges, and breastfeeding plays a crucial role in supporting the health and development of premature infants (Behrman, 2007). The benefits of breast milk are particularly vital for these babies, who are more vulnerable to infections and have underdeveloped organs (Alotiby, 2023).

Preterm breast milk is uniquely tailored to meet the specific needs of premature infants. It is higher in protein and contains more antibodies, supporting the development of the baby's immune system. The composition of breast milk changes dynamically, adapting to the changing nutritional needs of preterm infants as they grow and develop outside the womb.

One of the challenges faced by mothers of premature infants is the initial inability to breastfeed directly. In many cases, these babies are too small or medically fragile to latch onto the breast (Palmér& Ericson, 2019). However, mothers are encouraged to express breast milk using a breast pump, which can then be fed to the infant through a tube or bottle. This practice, known as expressing or pumping, ensures that premature infants still receive the invaluable benefits of breast milk even if they cannot nurse directly.

In addition to providing essential nutrients, breastfeeding helps create a bond between the mother and the premature infant, promoting emotional well-being for both. Kangaroo care, where the infant is held skin-to-skin on the mother's chest, is also beneficial for premature babies, promoting warmth, comfort, and stability.

Maternal health issues and breastfeeding

Some mothers may face health issues that complicate the breastfeeding journey. Conditions such as diabetes, hypertension, or infections may pose challenges, but in many cases, with proper support and guidance, breastfeeding can still be a viable option.

For mothers with diabetes, breastfeeding helps regulate blood sugar levels and reduces the risk of developing type 2 diabetes later in life (Alotiby, 2023). Breastfeeding also aids in weight loss after pregnancy, which is particularly beneficial for mothers with gestational diabetes.

In cases where the mother is HIV-positive, guidelines recommend exclusive breastfeeding with antiretroviral therapy to reduce the risk of transmission to the infant (Nlend, 2022). Breastfeeding, when managed with appropriate medical guidance, can still be a safe and viable option in such circumstances.

Breastfeeding with medical conditions in infants

Some infants are born with medical conditions that require special attention, and breastfeeding can be a key component of their care. For example, infants with cleft lip or palate may face challenges latching onto the breast, but with the support of healthcare professionals, mothers can still breastfeed successfully (Pathumwiwatana et al., 2010).

Breastfeeding is especially crucial for infants with congenital heart defects or other chronic conditions. The unique composition of breast milk provides the necessary nutrients without putting additional strain on the infant's delicate system. In some cases, breastfeeding may be recommended even if other medical interventions are necessary, as it offers additional comfort and support to the infant (Ford et al., 2020).

Breastfeeding in the neonatal intensive care unit (NICU)

Many infants with special health needs spend time in the Neonatal Intensive Care Unit (NICU). Breastfeeding in the NICU can be challenging due to the medical interventions and monitoring devices that these infants may require. However, healthcare professionals recognize the importance of breast milk for NICU babies and work closely with mothers to facilitate breastfeeding in such environments.

Mothers of NICU babies often face emotional stress and uncertainty, but the act of breastfeeding, even if initially through pumping, can provide a sense of connection and empowerment (Wang et al., 2021). NICU staff members are trained to support mothers in expressing and storing breast milk, ensuring that even the tiniest infants receive the benefits of their mother's milk.

Overcoming challenges: Lactation consultants and support groups

Addressing the challenges of breastfeeding in special circumstances requires a multidisciplinary approach. Lactation consultants play a pivotal role in guiding mothers through the process, offering expertise on techniques such as pumping, latching, and ensuring an adequate milk supply.

Support groups for mothers facing similar circumstances provide a valuable network for sharing experiences, tips, and emotional support. These groups can be in-person or online, allowing mothers to connect and find solace in the shared journey of breastfeeding in special circumstances.

The significance of breastfeeding in special circumstances

Breastfeeding in special circumstances is not just about providing nutrition; it's about offering a lifeline to vulnerable infants and creating a strong foundation for their health and development. The unique composition of breast milk, with its antibodies, immune-boosting factors, and tailored nutrition, becomes even more critical in these situations.

For mothers, breastfeeding is not only a physical act but also an emotional connection with their infants. It can be a source of comfort, empowerment, and resilience in the face of adversity. The act of nourishing their infants through breastfeeding, even when faced with challenges, reinforces the strength and determination of mothers in special circumstances.

Conclusions

Breastfeeding in special circumstances requires understanding, support, and a collaborative effort from healthcare professionals, families, and communities. While challenges may exist, the significance of breastfeeding in these situations cannot be overstated. It serves as a powerful tool in promoting the health and well-being of infants facing unique medical challenges and contributes to the emotional and physical recovery of mothers.

By recognizing the importance of breastfeeding in special circumstances and providing the necessary resources and support, we can ensure that all infants, regardless of their health circumstances, have the opportunity to benefit from the remarkable advantages that breast milk provides. Breastfeeding becomes not just a biological process but a testament to the strength, love, and resilience of both mothers and their infants.

References

1. Alotiby, A. (2023). The role of breastfeeding as a protective factor against the development of the immune-mediated diseases: A systematic review. Frontiers in Pediatrics, 11. https://doi.org/10.3389/fped.2023.1086999

2. Behrman, R. E. (2007). Mortality and acute complications in preterm infants. Preterm Birth - NCBI Bookshelf. https://www.ncbi.nlm.nih.gov/books/NBK11385/

3. Ford, E. L., Underwood, M. A., & German, J. B. (2020). Helping Mom Help Baby: Nutrition-Based Support for the Mother-Infant dyad during Lactation. Frontiers in Nutrition, 7. https://doi.org/10.3389/fnut.2020.00054

4. Nlend, A. E. N. (2022). Mother-to-Child Transmission of HIV Through Breastfeeding Improving Awareness and Education: A Short narrative review. International Journal of Women's Health, Volume 14, 697–703. https://doi.org/10.2147/ijwh.s330715

5. Palmér, L., & Ericson, J. (2019). A qualitative study on the breastfeeding experience of mothers of preterm infants in the first 12 months after birth. International Breastfeeding Journal, 14(1). https://doi.org/10.1186/s13006-019-0229-6

6. Pathumwiwatana, P., Tongsukho, S., Naratippakorn, T., Pradubwong, S., &Chusilp, K. (2010). The promotion of exclusive breastfeeding in infants with complete cleft lip and palate during the first 6 months after childbirth at Srinagarind Hospital, Khon Kaen Province, Thailand. PubMed, 93 Suppl 4, S71-7. https://pubmed.ncbi.nlm.nih.gov/21302391

7. Wang, L., Ma, J., Meng, H., & Jie, Z. (2021). Mothers' experiences of neonatal intensive care: A systematic review and implications for clinical practice. World Journal of Clinical Cases, 9(24), 7062–7072. https://doi.org/10.12998/wjcc.v9.i24.7062

15.

Enrichment in Women's Health through Nutrients: Nourishment, Healthyness and Breastfeeding

Dr. Pratibha S. Katkar

Head and Asst. Prof.

(Department of Home Economics)

Yeshwant Mahavidyalaya, Wardha

Email: pratibhavaidya82@gmail.com

Abstract

Nutrition is an important part of wellness and healing. Better nutrition has been identified as improving infant, youth and maternal well-being, a more grounded and safer environment, safer pregnancy and childbirth, lower risk of contracting non-communicable infections (such as diabetes and cardiovascular disease) and longer life expectancy. The issue of coping for women in agricultural countries is usually compared to the mother's diet, emphasizing the effect of the mother's health status on birth weight and during breastfeeding. The effect of maternal well-being and nutrition on performance has not been much considered in friendly and financial exercises. The cultural situation of India changed rapidly in terms of female education, and the financial commitment to the family became even stronger. Women take many parts that can affect their well-being because they are parental figures and today the family structure is changing to a more nuclear one. The work status of women is directly related to their social status. The well-being of a woman is an important consequence of the well-being of her offspring. Many women do not get enough time for self-care and also for young people, while they have more independence from the rat race than unemployed women due to forgetfulness, work stress or moving both at home and at work, and absenteeism. time [Monga S et al., 2008]. These lifestyles pushed by the general public have shifted more towards convenient food sources that are high in energy and fat.

Keywords: Women, health, food, nutrients, well-being, Breastfeeding.

Introduction

Healthy children learn better. People who get enough food are helpful and can slowly open doors to destroy needs and appetites. Lack of healthy nutrition in any structure is a huge threat to human well-being. Today, the world faces the double burden of hunger, which includes both malnutrition and obesity, especially in low- and middle-income countries. WHO provides sound advice and dynamic tools to help countries fight all forms of hunger to promote well-being and prosperity at all ages. This real-life documentary explores the dangers and reactions of all kinds of diseases starting at very specific stages of development, which the welfare framework can directly and indirectly influence in various areas, especially the food framework. The Importance of Women's and Girls' Participation in Public Efforts to Increase Nutrition As evidence has long shown, gender differences can play a role, as can the effects of appetite and hunger. Of course, greater differentiation between the sexes is associated with an increase in both acute and chronic malnutrition.3, Gender and livelihood are not independent issues for some experts who believe that women are the spheres of nutrition, well-being and nutrition.

Women nutrition

A solid, adjusted eating regimen is the foundation of driving a sound way of life for all kinds of people. As youngsters, young men and young ladies by and large need exactly the same things from their eating routine. However, as adolescence starts, carrying with it changes to the body and chemicals, ladies have diverse wholesome requirements from men.

Calorie utilization

The NHS suggests that the normal man and lady of sound weight ought to burn-through around 2,500kcal every day for men, and 2,000kcal per day for ladies. These qualities can, obviously, fluctuate contingent upon age, digestion and levels of active work, among other things.While everybody is unique and the quantity of calories you need will rely upon a few variables, as a general rule, ladies should devour less calories. In case you're hoping to acquire or get more fit, addressing your GP as well as a nourishment expert can assist you with seeing the number of calories you ought to be burning-through.

Dietary necessities for women

Just as requiring less calories than men, ladies have some unique dietary necessities from men. This is predominantly a result of the chemicals ladies produce.

The accompanying nutrients and minerals are especially critical to include:

Iron

At the point when ladies arrive at childbearing age, blood misfortune through feminine cycle can prompt iron lack or sickliness. Therefore, ladies will generally require more iron than men. Iron can be found in a scope of food sources, including meat, fish and poultry and non-creature items like spinach, lentils and strengthened grains. Nutrient C will assist your body with retaining more iron, so you ought to likewise hope to incorporate food sources that are plentiful in this nutrient, like broccoli, tomatoes and citrus natural products. Just as increasing your admission of iron-rich food sources and wellsprings of nutrient C, think about your present eating regimen and what could be diminished. Healthful advisor Claire Hargreaves (BSc Hons) examines what your every day tea or espresso could be meaning for your degrees of iron.

Calcium

Each individual requirements least 2 liters of water ordinary. Having diet rich food isn't adequate. Likewise having the food at the ideal opportunity matters a great deal. Skipping breakfast or lunch is anything but a smart thought. For grown-ups ideal time for supper ought to be 7 pm. Yet, working ladies might think that it is troublesome. So they can have light food varieties like plates of mixed greens or soups for supper. They can select weighty breakfast toward the beginning of the day. Food with a lot of salt or sugar ought to be kept away from to forestall hazard of hypertension and diabetes. It is smarter to remember 2 servings of natural products for a day. However, it isn't prudent to eat the two organic products together. Its is a great idea to have 3 major dinners and 5 little suppers for solid digestion and keeping up with weight.

Vegan working Women

Vegan diets can be sound. However, having a fair eating regimen requires some additional consideration. By eating an assortment of food sources including natural products, vegetables, vegetables, nuts and seeds, soy items, and entire grains, vegans can get sufficient supplements from non–meat sources.

- Vegetarians ought to make certain to eat an assortment of entire grains like entire wheat bread, pasta and tortillas, earthy colored rice, oats, bulgur, and quinoa.

- For the solid body, fats are likewise required. Solid fats incorporate nuts or nut margarines, oils, and avocados

- Nuts, nut spreads, soy food varieties, beans, peas, dairy food sources like milk, yogurt, and cheddar and eggs all give great protein.

- Include figs and apricots in your morning meal and bites to keep away from iron lack. Green leaves like spinach additionally helps for this.

Nutrition during and after childbirth (this is the type of food women should eat before and after childbirth) your body's health needs increase during pregnancy. Most pregnant women can meet these broader nutritional needs by choosing a nutritional routine that includes a variety of high-quality foods. Cereals are a good source of energy. Foods grown from the ground are full of cancer-preventing agents, fiber, and water- and fat-soluble nutrients. Foods that include meat, nuts and vegetables provide your body with protein, folate and iron. Dairy products are the best source of calcium and dietary D. There should be at least 3 months of vacation. In a perfect world, you would need half a year off to fully recover. It is basically for baby. During these six months, the child needs the mother the most. Also, if the mother stops breastfeeding after 3 months, the child may develop contamination such as ear diseases due to low sensitivity.

Fitness through physical activities

The participation of women in sports increased in the second half of the 20th century, and on July 23, 1972, another March 8 dawned, this time in sports. US President Nixon signed the famous Title IX (Education Amendment Act), which states that No one in the

United States shall be excluded, hindered or discriminated against on the basis of sex in any educational program or publicly funded activity. (Michel) and Ennis, 2007). The number of scholarships awarded since the signing of Title IX through the 1980s. and thus the proportion of active sportswomen increased by 700% and another 50% in the 90s. At the beginning of the new millennium, every third American high school student was actively involved in sports, in 1972 every 27 (Iirimaa and Ott, 200). London 2012 saw another record with a record number of participants, 6% of the more than 10,000 participants, compared to a male ratio of 53:1 in 1908. Sports offer advantages to men over women. Girls who play sports do better in school, have fewer unwanted teenage pregnancies, have higher self-esteem and confidence, get into colleges and universities more easily and more often, and have fewer problems. with substance abuse and addiction disorders. Bodyweight training has immeasurable benefits for developing and maintaining bone mass in women of all ages (Hagen, 2005). Nature, however, did not sign the declaration on gender equality in sport. When it comes to physical activity, it has long been said that women are the "weaker sex". Not only can all sports be played in the name of gender equality, it results in women developing many of the developmental characteristics characteristic of men. According to Nikola Grujic, biology has already distinguished between the sexes during development, especially according to their reproductive roles, so that "messing up in their affairs" has unpredictable consequences, the price of which is in any case very expensive.

Importance of breastfeeding for better health

Breastfeeding has health benefits for both babies and mothers. Breast milk provides a baby with ideal nutrition and supports growth and development. Breastfeeding can also help protect baby and mom against certain illnesses and diseases.

Five great benefits of breastfeeding

1. **Breast milk is the best source of nutrition for most babies:** As the baby grows, the mother's breast milk will change to meet the baby's nutritional needs.

2. **Breastfeeding can help protect babies against some short- and long-term illnesses and diseases:** Breastfed babies have a lower risk of asthma, obesity, type 1 diabetes, and sudden infant death syndrome (SIDS). Breastfed babies are also less likely to have ear infections and stomach bugs.

3. **Breast milk shares antibodies from the mother with her baby:** These antibodies help babies develop a strong immune system and protect them from illnesses.

4. **Mothers can breastfeed anytime and anywhere:** Mothers can feed their babies on the go without worrying about having to mix formula or prepare bottles.

When travelling breastfeeding can also provide a source of comfort for babies whose normal routine is disrupted.

5. **Breastfeeding can reduce the mother's risk of breast and ovarian cancer, type 2 diabetes, and high blood pressure:** Breastfeeding has health benefits for the mother too! Some cancers, type 2 diabetes, and high blood pressure are less common among women who breastfeed.

Conclusions

There are many variables to think about while keeping a solid eating regimen. Our bodies are continually changing for the duration of our lives, so we can't anticipate following a similar eating routine arrangement all through our lifetime - as we've investigated, our nourishing requirements change. That, however our food inclinations change as well. To appreciate food, suppers should be fluctuated and fascinating. Thinking about these components, it tends to be hard to concoct a solid eating routine arrangement ourselves.

References

1. "Malignant growth Prevention During Early Life | CDC". www.cdc.gov. 2020-07-14. Recovered 2020-10-29.

2. Barasi EM (2003). Human Nutrition - A Health Perspective. London: Arnold. ISBN 978-0-340-81025-5.

3.	"WHO | 10 realities on sustenance". World Health Organization. 2011-03-15. Recovered 2011-08-07.

4.	Riley L (2006). Pregnancy: The Ultimate Week-by-Week Pregnancy Guide. Meredith Books. pp. 21–22. ISBN 978-0-696-22221-4.

5.	Starling, Phoebe; Charlton, Karen; McMahon, Anne T.; Lucas, Catherine (2015-03-18). "Fish Intake during Pregnancy and Fetal Neurodevelopment—A Systematic Review of the Evidence". Supplements. 7 (3): 2001–2014. doi:10.3390/nu7032001. PMC 4377896. PMID 25793632

16.

Breastfeeding Unveiled: Myths, Food, Barriers and Addressing Milk Supply Cessation

Surbhee Gupta

Assistant at LIC of India

Email: sb7529@gmail.com

Misconceptions related to breastfeeding

Misconceptions related to breastfeeding are common and can lead to misunderstandings or barriers to successful breastfeeding. It's essential to address these misconceptions to provide accurate information and support to mothers.

Misconception: "I don't have enough milk."

Many mothers worry that their milk supply is insufficient. However, most mothers produce enough milk for their baby's needs, and the baby's feeding cues, rather than the amount of milk expressed, are the best indicator of sufficiency.

Misconception: "Breastfeeding is painful."

While some discomfort or tenderness may occur initially, breastfeeding should not be painful. Pain can be a sign of an improper latch or other issues that need to be addressed with proper support and guidance.

Misconception: "Formula is just as good as breast milk."

Breast milk is uniquely tailored to a baby's nutritional and immune needs. It contains antibodies, live cells, and various bioactive components that formula cannot replicate. Breastfeeding provides health benefits for both the baby and mother.

Misconception: "Breastfeeding ruins the shape of breasts."

Breastfeeding does not inherently alter breast shape. Changes in breast appearance can occur with pregnancy, weight fluctuations, or the natural aging process, but breastfeeding alone is not a major factor.

Misconception: "Babies should be on a strict feeding schedule."

Breastfed babies should be fed on demand, following their cues for hunger. Rigid schedules can hinder milk production and responsiveness to the baby's needs.

Misconception: "Breastfeeding interferes with birth control."

While breastfeeding can provide some natural contraception (known as the lactational amenorrhea method), it is not foolproof. Mothers should use a reliable birth control method if they wish to prevent pregnancy while breastfeeding.

Misconception: "I should avoid certain foods while breastfeeding."

In most cases, breastfeeding mothers can enjoy a varied diet. While some babies may be sensitive to certain foods, there is no need for mothers to avoid entire food groups unless advised by a healthcare provider.

Misconception: "I can't breastfeed if I'm sick."

In many cases, mothers can continue breastfeeding when they are ill, as breast milk provides antibodies that can benefit the baby's immune system. Consultation with a healthcare provider can guide decisions on breastfeeding during illness.

Misconception: "Breastfeeding prevents babies from sleeping through the night."

Babies have different sleep patterns, and some may wake during the night for feeding even if they are breastfed. However, breastfeeding itself is not a cause of disrupted sleep patterns.

Misconception: "Breastfeeding is only for the first few months."

The World Health Organization recommends exclusive breastfeeding for the first six months and continued breastfeeding with complementary foods for up to two years or longer. Breastfeeding can provide ongoing health benefits.

Addressing these misconceptions with accurate information and providing breastfeeding education and support can empower mothers to make informed choices and promote successful and fulfilling breastfeeding experiences.

Foods that hindered the breast milk supply

While many foods are safe to consume while breastfeeding, some foods and substances may potentially hinder milk supply or cause sensitivity in some infants. It's important to note that individual reactions can vary, and not all breastfeeding mothers will be affected by these foods. Here are some foods and substances that some mothers find may have an impact on breast milk supply or their baby's comfort:

Sage and peppermint

These herbs, especially in concentrated forms like essential oils, have been associated with a decrease in milk supply. Consuming them in normal culinary amounts, such as seasoning in food, is generally considered safe.

Caffeine

Excessive caffeine intake can affect some babies' sleep patterns and cause fussiness. While moderate caffeine consumption is typically fine for most breastfeeding mothers, excessive caffeine intake should be avoided.

Alcohol

Alcohol can pass into breast milk, potentially affecting the baby's sleep and development. It's best to limit alcohol consumption and allow sufficient time for alcohol to metabolize before breastfeeding.

Cabbage and peppermint tea

Some mothers believe that consuming large amounts of cabbage or drinking peppermint tea can decrease milk supply. These foods are generally safe in moderation, but excessive consumption may have an impact on supply.

High-mercury fish

Certain fish, like shark, swordfish, king mackerel, and tilefish, can contain high levels of mercury, which can be harmful to a baby's developing nervous system. Choose fish lower in mercury, such as salmon, sardines, and trout.

Spicy foods

Spicy foods can sometimes cause gastrointestinal discomfort in babies, leading to fussiness or gas. Some babies may be more sensitive to spices than others.

Dairy products (in cases of lactose intolerance)

If a baby is lactose intolerant, dairy products in the mother's diet can potentially lead to discomfort in the baby. In such cases, the mother may need to eliminate dairy temporarily and consult a healthcare provider for guidance.

Gas-producing vegetables

Certain vegetables like broccoli, cauliflower, and beans can produce gas in some infants, leading to gassiness or fussiness. Again, individual reactions vary, and not all babies are affected.

Allergenic foods (in rare cases)

In some instances, babies may exhibit sensitivity or allergy to certain foods in the mother's diet, such as cow's milk, nuts, or eggs. If there are concerns about allergies, consult a healthcare provider for guidance.

It's important for breastfeeding mothers to pay attention to their own diet and their baby's reactions. If you suspect that a specific food is causing discomfort or a decrease in milk supply, it may be helpful to keep a food diary and gradually eliminate or reintroduce foods while monitoring your baby's response. If you have concerns about your breast milk supply or your baby's reactions to your diet, it's advisable to consult a lactation consultant or healthcare provider for guidance and support.

Barriers of breast feeding

Breastfeeding is widely recognized as the optimal way to nourish infants due to its numerous health benefits. However, various barriers can hinder breastfeeding initiation and duration. These barriers can be categorized into several key areas:

Lack of knowledge and education

Misconceptions: Myths and misconceptions about breastfeeding can discourage mothers. For example, some may believe that they don't produce enough milk or that breastfeeding is painful.

Inadequate education: A lack of information and education on breastfeeding can leave mothers feeling unprepared and unsure about how to breastfeed effectively.

Cultural and societal factors

Cultural beliefs: Cultural norms and beliefs may promote or discourage breastfeeding. Some cultures may have taboos or traditions that hinder breastfeeding.

Social stigma: Negative attitudes towards breastfeeding in public can make mothers uncomfortable nursing in public spaces.

Lack of family support: Lack of support from family members, especially partners, can be a significant barrier.

Workplace and employment

Inadequate maternity leave: Limited or unpaid maternity leave can force mothers to return to work before they are ready, making it challenging to continue breastfeeding.

Lack of pumping facilities: Insufficient access to clean and private spaces for pumping breast milk at the workplace can discourage working mothers from continuing to breastfeed.

Inflexible Work Schedules: Inflexible work hours may not allow for breaks for breastfeeding or pumping.

Healthcare practices and support

Inadequate prenatal education: Some healthcare providers may not provide enough information on breastfeeding during prenatal care visits.

Lack of postpartum support: Mothers may face difficulties with breastfeeding in the early postpartum period due to insufficient guidance or lactation support.

Inaccurate medical advice: Healthcare professionals who lack proper training in lactation may inadvertently provide incorrect advice.

Medical and physical challenges

Maternal health issues: Certain maternal health conditions, such as breast surgery or certain medications, can make breastfeeding difficult or contraindicated.

Infant health issues: Prematurity, tongue-tie, or other medical conditions in infants can pose breastfeeding challenges.

Pain and discomfort: Some women experience pain, nipple issues, or engorgement, which can affect their breastfeeding experience.

Marketing and promotion of formula milk

Aggressive marketing: Aggressive marketing of infant formula by formula companies can influence mothers' decisions to formula-feed.

Free formula samples: The distribution of free formula samples in hospitals or through marketing campaigns can undermine breastfeeding.

Lack of access to lactation support

Limited access to lactation consultants: Many mothers may not have access to lactation consultants or support groups, which can be essential for addressing breastfeeding challenges.

Cost barriers: The cost of lactation support services can be prohibitive for some families.

Public policy and legal barriers

Lack of legal protections: Some regions lack legal protections for breastfeeding mothers, including laws supporting breastfeeding in public spaces or at the workplace.

Insufficient parental leave policies: Limited parental leave policies can hinder mothers' ability to establish and maintain breastfeeding.

Addressing these barriers requires a multi-faceted approach · involving healthcare professionals, policymakers, employers, families, and communities. Supportive policies, increased education, and improved access to lactation support can help more mothers initiate and continue breastfeeding, promoting the health and well-being of both infants and mothers.

Factors associated with cessation of exclusive breastfeeding

Several factors can be associated with the cessation of exclusive breastfeeding before the recommended duration of six months. These factors are often interrelated and can vary among individuals and communities.

Maternal employment

Returning to work can make it challenging for mothers to continue exclusive breastfeeding. The lack of adequate maternity leave or flexible work hours can force mothers to introduce formula or complementary foods earlier.

Perceived insufficient milk supply

Many mothers may believe they have an insufficient milk supply due to concerns about infant hunger or weight gain. This perception can lead to early introduction of formula or complementary foods.

Breastfeeding challenges

Difficulties with latching, nipple pain, engorgement, or other breastfeeding challenges can lead to frustration and early weaning if not addressed with proper support and guidance.

Cultural and social norms

Cultural beliefs and societal norms may encourage the introduction of complementary foods at an early age. Family and peer pressure can influence a mother's decision to cease exclusive breastfeeding.

Lack of knowledge and education

Mothers who are not well-informed about the benefits of exclusive breastfeeding and the recommended duration may not realize the importance of continuing it until six months.

Marketing of formula milk

Aggressive marketing of infant formula can influence mothers' decisions to use formula. The distribution of free formula samples in hospitals or through marketing campaigns can undermine breastfeeding.

Perceived convenience

Some mothers may perceive formula feeding as more convenient, especially if they have concerns about breastfeeding in public or managing breastfeeding while working.

Family and peer support

Lack of support from family members, especially partners, can be a significant factor. Supportive family members and friends can encourage and enable mothers to continue exclusive breastfeeding.

Healthcare practices

Inadequate support and guidance from healthcare providers during pregnancy, childbirth, and the postpartum period can contribute to early cessation of exclusive breastfeeding.

Breastfeeding knowledge and confidence

A mother's confidence in her ability to breastfeed successfully can impact her decision to continue exclusive breastfeeding. Lack of confidence may lead to the introduction of complementary foods or formula.

Early introduction of complementary foods

Introducing solid foods before six months of age can lead to early cessation of exclusive breastfeeding. Some caregivers may mistakenly believe that the baby needs solid foods for adequate nutrition.

Maternal health issues

Maternal health conditions, such as medication use or illnesses, can sometimes necessitate the cessation of breastfeeding earlier than desired.

Infant health issues

Health issues or concerns related to the infant's growth or development can prompt caregivers to introduce formula or complementary foods earlier.

Access to healthcare and support services

Access to lactation consultants, support groups, and healthcare services can impact a mother's ability to address breastfeeding challenges and continue exclusive breastfeeding.

To promote exclusive breastfeeding for the recommended duration of six months, healthcare providers, communities, and policymakers should work together to address these factors. Providing comprehensive education, lactation support, workplace accommodations, and promoting a breastfeeding-friendly culture can help mothers make informed choices and successfully continue exclusive breastfeeding.

17

Breastmilk Supply and Galactogogs

Archana Gupta

Homemaker,

Kota Rajasthan

Reasons of low supply of breastmilk

Low breast milk supply is a concern for some breastfeeding mothers and can be attributed to various factors. It's important to note that many mothers can successfully increase their milk supply with proper support and strategies.

Inadequate breast stimulation

Effective breastfeeding relies on proper latch and frequent, effective milk removal. If the baby does not latch well or feed frequently enough, it can lead to low milk supply.

Infrequent feedings

Babies need frequent feedings, especially in the early weeks of life. Infrequent feedings can signal to the body that less milk is needed, potentially leading to decreased supply.

Poor latch

An improper latch can prevent the baby from effectively removing milk from the breast. This can occur due to issues such as tongue-tie, lip-tie, or a shallow latch.

Supplementing with formula

Offering formula supplementation in addition to breastfeeding can reduce the demand for breast milk, signaling to the body to produce less milk.

Pacifier and bottle use

Introducing pacifiers or bottles too early can lead to nipple confusion, making it difficult for the baby to latch effectively and feed at the breast.

Maternal stress and anxiety

High levels of stress and anxiety can interfere with the letdown reflex and milk production. It's essential for mothers to find ways to manage stress effectively.

Medical conditions

Certain medical conditions, such as polycystic ovary syndrome (PCOS), hormonal imbalances, thyroid disorders, or insufficient glandular tissue, can affect milk production.

Previous breast surgeries

Breast surgeries, including reductions or augmentations, can disrupt milk ducts and glandular tissue, potentially impacting milk production.

Medications

Some medications, including certain birth control pills, decongestants, or antihistamines, can suppress milk production. It's important to consult with a healthcare provider if taking medications while breastfeeding.

Breastfeeding on a schedule

Instead of feeding on demand, following a rigid feeding schedule may not allow for frequent enough milk removal, potentially decreasing supply.

Premature birth

Babies born prematurely may have difficulty breastfeeding initially, which can affect milk production. In such cases, pumping and providing expressed milk can help.

Inadequate hydration and nutrition

Proper maternal hydration and nutrition are essential for milk production. A well-balanced diet and staying adequately hydrated are crucial.

Weaning too soon

If a mother starts weaning her baby off the breast before the baby is ready, it can lead to decreased milk supply.

It's important to remember that many cases of perceived low milk supply can be addressed and improved with the right support and strategies. Working with a lactation consultant or healthcare provider can help identify the underlying cause and develop a plan to increase milk supply if needed.

Techniques like frequent breastfeeding or pumping, proper latch and positioning, skin-to-skin contact, and managing maternal stress can be effective in boosting milk production.

Factors improving breast milk supply

Improving breast milk supply can often be achieved with the right strategies and support. If you're concerned about your milk supply, consider trying the following methods:

Frequent and effective nursing

Ensure that your baby is latching properly and nursing effectively. Frequent breastfeeding stimulates milk production. Offer the breast whenever your baby shows hunger cues.

Breast compression

While nursing, use breast compression to encourage milk flow. Gently squeeze your breast as the baby feeds to help them get more milk.

Skin-to-skin contact

Spend time with your baby in skin-to-skin contact, which can enhance bonding and stimulate milk production.

Empty the breasts

Allow your baby to nurse on one breast until it's emptied before switching to the other breast. This helps ensure that your baby receives both the foremilk (thinner, hydrating milk) and hindmilk (richer, calorie-dense milk).

Cluster feeding

Some babies go through cluster feeding periods where they want to nurse frequently over a short period. Allow this, as it can help increase your milk supply.

Pump after feeds

If your baby doesn't fully empty the breast, pump for a few minutes after nursing to signal to your body that more milk is needed.

Breast massage

Gentle breast massage before or during nursing can help improve milk flow.

Stay hydrated and well-nourished

Drink plenty of water and consume a balanced diet. Being well-hydrated and properly nourished is essential for milk production.

Rest and self-care

Get adequate rest and manage stress. Fatigue and stress can negatively impact milk supply.

Galactagogues

Some herbs and foods are believed to boost milk supply. Fenugreek, fennel, and oatmeal are examples. Consult with a healthcare provider or lactation consultant before using galactagogues.

Medication

In some cases, medication may be prescribed to increase milk supply. Discuss this option with your healthcare provider.

Seek lactation support

Consult with a lactation consultant or breastfeeding specialist for guidance and personalized strategies to increase milk supply.

Avoid unnecessary supplements

If your healthcare provider hasn't recommended it, avoid using formula supplements, as they can decrease your milk supply by reducing the demand for breastfeeding.

Breastfeed on demand

Respond promptly to your baby's hunger cues rather than following a strict feeding schedule.

Avoid pacifiers and bottles early on

Delay introducing pacifiers and bottles until breastfeeding is well-established to prevent nipple confusion.

Evaluate medications and birth control

Some medications and birth control methods can affect milk supply. Discuss these with your healthcare provider.

Remember that it may take a few days to see an increase in milk supply when implementing these strategies. Be patient with yourself, and seek support from healthcare professionals or support groups if needed. Every mother's breastfeeding journey is unique, and there are often solutions to improve milk supply when challenges arise.

Galactogogs

Galactagogues, often referred to as "galactogogs," are substances that are believed to help increase milk production in breastfeeding mothers. These substances can include herbs, foods, and medications. It's important to note that while some women may find galactagogues helpful, their effectiveness can vary, and their use should be discussed with a healthcare provider or lactation consultant. Here are some common galactagogues:

Fenugreek

Fenugreek seeds are a well-known galactagogue. They can be consumed in various forms, including as a supplement, tea, or spice in cooking.

Fennel

Fennel seeds and fennel tea are often used to support milk production. Some mothers consume fennel seeds directly, while others prefer fennel tea.

Brewer's yeast

Brewer's yeast is rich in B vitamins and can be added to foods like smoothies or lactation cookies to potentially boost milk supply.

Oatmeal

Oats are a source of complex carbohydrates and fiber. Many nursing mothers find that eating oatmeal in various forms, such as oatmeal cookies or porridge, can support milk production.

Alfalfa

Alfalfa is often taken in the form of supplements or herbal tea. It is believed to have galactogenic properties.

Blessed thistle

Blessed thistle is an herb that is sometimes used in combination with fenugreek to enhance its galactogenic effects.

Goat's rue

Goat's rue is another herbal supplement that some mothers use to increase milk supply.

Pumpkin seeds

Some women believe that pumpkin seeds can help support milk production. They can be consumed as a snack or added to various dishes.

Shatavari

Shatavari is an herb used in traditional Ayurvedic medicine and is sometimes considered a galactagogue.

Malunggay (moringa)

Malunggay leaves, often known as moringa leaves, are rich in nutrients and are used as a galactagogue in some cultures.

It's important to exercise caution when using galactagogues. While many of these substances are generally considered safe for consumption, they may not be suitable for everyone, and their effectiveness can vary from person to person. If you're considering using galactagogues to increase your milk supply, it's advisable to consult with a healthcare provider or a lactation consultant who can provide guidance tailored to your specific situation. Additionally, it's essential to maintain a well-balanced diet, stay hydrated, and ensure proper breastfeeding techniques for optimal milk production.

Should a new mother use galactogogs

Whether a new mother should use galactagogues (substances believed to increase milk supply) depends on her individual circumstances and needs. It's important to approach the use of galactagogues with caution and consider the following factors:

Consultation with healthcare provider

Before using galactagogues, it's crucial for a new mother to consult with her healthcare provider, preferably a lactation consultant or a healthcare professional experienced in breastfeeding. They can assess her specific situation and provide personalized guidance.

Evaluation of milk supply

Determining if there is a true issue with milk supply is essential. Sometimes perceived low supply can be improved with adjustments to breastfeeding techniques, latch, frequency, and other factors.

Potential underlying causes

If there is a concern about milk supply, it's essential to address any potential underlying causes, such as latch issues, infrequent feedings, or stress, before turning to galactagogues.

Safety and side effects

Some galactagogues may have side effects or interact with medications the mother is taking. Discuss the safety and potential risks of using galactagogues with a healthcare provider.

Non-pharmacological approaches

Non-pharmacological methods to increase milk supply, such as frequent breastfeeding, skin-to-skin contact, and ensuring proper latch and positioning, should be explored and encouraged first.

Balanced diet and hydration

A nutritious diet and proper hydration are essential for milk production. Ensuring the mother is well-nourished and adequately hydrated is a fundamental step.

Mother's preferences and comfort

The decision to use galactagogues should also consider the mother's comfort and preferences. Some mothers may prefer non-pharmacological methods, while others may be open to trying galactagogues.

Medications

If considering prescription galactagogues like domperidone or metoclopramide, these should only be used under the supervision and recommendation of a healthcare provider.

Monitoring and adjustments

If galactagogues are used, it's important to monitor their effectiveness and be prepared to adjust the approach if necessary.

Breastfeeding goals

A mother's goals for breastfeeding should be taken into account. If she is committed to exclusively breastfeeding, she may explore galactagogues more readily than if she is supplementing with formula.

In summary, the decision to use galactagogues should be made on an individual basis, with input from a healthcare provider who can assess the mother's specific situation and needs. It's essential to explore non-pharmacological methods first and prioritize the well-being of both the mother and the baby. Effective breastfeeding support and guidance are key to addressing any concerns about milk supply.

List of Published Books

1. Gupta K and Jain M. Vridhopayogi Vyanjan: Vridhjano ke liye Upcharatmak Pak Vidhiyan. Abhinav Prakashan. Ajmer. 2016. ISBN: 978-938418946-4

This book contains more than 65 healthy food recipes developed, prepared and clinically verified by myself alone, tailored with the nutritional needs of the geriatric population.

2. Gupta K. Community Science and Sustainable Community Development. Lambart Academic Publication. Germany 2021. ISBN: 978-620419757-9

This book provides excellent research data related to different aspects of community which will be helpful to strengthen the sustainability of a community in terms of health, nutrition, wellness and economy.

3. Gupta K. 75 years of Indian Independence: Food and Nutritional Achievements, Opportunities and Challenges (Volume 1). Notion Press. Chennai. 2022. ISBN: 979-888883053-6

4. Gupta K. 75 years of Indian Independence: Food and Nutritional Achievements, Opportunities and Challenges (Volume 2). Notion Press. Chennai. 2022. ISBN: 979-888883757-3

5. Gupta K. 75 years of Indian Independence: Food and Nutritional Achievements, Opportunities and Challenges (Volume 3). Notion Press. Chennai. 2022. ISBN: 979-888909005-2

These three books provide enriched research data pertaining to various aspects of health, lifestyle, tourism, agriculture, antenatal or post natal diet, nutritional status, cognition and nutrition, etc., that will be extremely helpful to improve quality of life of the individuals ultimately making healthy and sustainable community.

6. Gupta K. Aazadi ka Amrit Mahotsav: Community Science Achievements, Opportunities and Challenges. BlueRose One Publishers. India. 2023. ISBN: 978-935704938-2

This book is particularly based on different disciplines of community science, i.e., food science and nutrition, food security, advancement in food preservation and processing, sustainable breeding and cultivation approaches in agriculture, importance of prebiotics, role of therapeutic diet, importance of nutrition for pregnant ladies and children, how cognitive development is affected by nutritional status of the children, spiritual development, skill based learning system DEASA, effect of social media on community development.

7. Gupta K. Nutrition Education: An Important Pillar of Health. Notion Press. Chennai. 2023. ISBN: 979-888959915-9

This book is particularly based on different topics of nutrition science, i.e., importance of nutrition in daily life, flavours of Bengal, flavours of Ramadan, Indian spices, celebrate a world of flavours, nutrition in bed bound patients, why nutrition is essential and importance of homemade pickles in daily diet.

8. Gupta K, Bhushan V, Pandey A. Issues with Girls. Notion Press. Chennai. 2023. ISBN: 979-889026221-9

This book is particularly based on different topics related to girls and women, i.e., change in education to bring empowerment, mental hygiene, health and diet management, rise in health problems: A wake up call, girls hygiene and nutrients, letting the girls grow naturally, nutrition for girls, optimal nutrition, good health and wellbeing,: are we there yet?, women's leadership and role model for girls, empowering girls: dare to dream, baby girl: beautiful miracles.

9. Gupta K, Tripathi KM, Meena N, Sukhwal I, Soni V. Recent Trends in Community Science. BlueRose One Publishers. India. 2023. ISBN: 978-935819026-7

This book is based on different area of community science, i.e., parenting techniques and changes in parenting over the time, association between eating out and childhood obesity, rural participation and community development, ergonomics for everyone, kitchen ergonomics, use of unconventional fibres in textile industry, sustainable techniques for dye application (textile industry), spiritual development, therapeutic nutrition, impact of dietary habits on people suffering from polycystic ovarian syndrome (PCOS), millets: heritage of India, *terminalia arjuna* herb and its impact on hypercholesterolemia's patients, black cumin seeds, development disorders of children and homoeopathic treatment, success stories of women entrepreneurs from fields of community science.

10. Gupta K, Katiyar P, Meena S, Tripathi KM,. Millets: The Miracle of Nature. Notion Press. Chennai. 2023. ISBN: 979-889066606-2

This book is particularly based on topics such as millets- the nutria-cereal, magical grains, millets- the climate resilient nutria cereals, India's treasury: millets as dietary accessory, therapeutic role of millets in daily life, nutritional impact of millets on pregnant mothers, economic aspects of millets etc,.

11. Gupta K, Cherian B, Ramalakshmi, Harjai K. Health and Wellness (A basic guide to obtain good health). Notion Press. Chennai. 2023. ISBN: 979-889067222-3

Chapters of this book entitled "Health and Wellness (A basic guide to obtain good health)" particularly based on topics such as Blood, breathing & thoughts, Meditation, yoga, silence and prayer, Mind-body connection: Using yoga to enhance maternal health, Improve your low self-esteem with blessings of yoga and meditation, Food habits, Nutrition for health, Biogreens: the immunity booster, Role of nutrition in obesity, No health without mental health, Ayurveda for holistic health care, Homoeopathic biochemic treatment, Palliative care, Functional foods in cardiovascular disease, Union government initiatives to provide affordable, accessible, and quality healthcare for all.

12. Gupta K, Gaur V, Kumari R, Mishra S, Arya L, Mukharjee G. Health for All. Notion Press. Chennai. 2023. ISBN: 979-889133024-5

The edited book volume is primarily intended to be a collection of peer reviewed and plagiarism free chapters written by research scholars, academicians, scientists, doctors and faculty members of their respective fields. Chapters of this book entitled "Health for All" particularly based on topics such as sustainable innovation strategies in public health, application of technology in healthcare, world health organization's policies on world nutrition, the invisible threat of food borne diseases, obesity in affluent societies and its effect, role of nutrition education, treatment of diseases using different medical systems, non communicable diseases through workplace wellness initiatives, immunization program and serum banking in India.

13. Gupta K, Swamy D, Jain S, Sangeeta, Rochani C, Verma R. Current Advances in Community Science. Notion Press. Chennai. 2023. ISBN: 979-8891186087-2

The edited book volume is primarily intended to be a collection of peer reviewed and plagiarism free chapters particularly based on topics such as impact and benefits of nano-fertilizers, understanding the benefits of dietary fibres on health, importance of food fortification, consumer problems and protection in India related to adulteration, black marketing, health and psychological well-being, role of millets to sustain food and nutritional security, extension education in modern era, paradigm shift in extension approaches for sustainable development, computer aided designing in textiles and apparel industry, use of microfibers, Instagram as a tool to promote micro apparels and qualitative analysis on the different areas of skill development in community science.

14. Gupta K, Katiyar P, Verma P, Pawar RV, Sangeeta. Food Safety & Security- A Basic Guide. Notion Press. Chennai. 2023. ISBN: 979-889233007-7

Chapters of this book entitled "Food safety and food security (A basic guide)" particularly based on topics such as foodborne diseases, immunity boosters, feeding the nation, when food turns foul, national and international organizations working for food safety, food spoilage, food poisoning, food preservation, food safety, food security, food safety and standard authority of India (FSSAI), natural farming, food standards, food safety risk assessment and management, role of government in ensuring food safety, role of food pickles in achieving household food security, assessing the benefits and costs of improving food safety.

15. Gupta K, Venkatappa KG, Devi KV, Sangeeta, Pal P. Brain: Associations, Wellness & Treatment. Notion Press. Chennai. 2024. ISBN: 979-889233671-0

Chapters of this book entitled **"Brain: Associations, Wellness and Treatment"** particularly based on topics such as brain health and disabilities, what I learnt about our brain, heads off to migraine, effect of stress on mental health, unlocking mental wellness, Parkinson's disease and its homeopathic treatment, mental health, depression, interrelation between brain health and cognitive functioning, artificial intelligence and cognitive science, effect of sleep patterns on brain health, prioritizing brain health, spirituality and brain health, impact of financial condition on brain heath, drugs and brain health; and impact of homemade food on maintaining brain health and wellness.

16. Gupta K, Mukharjee G, Esaivani KB, Sangeeta, Anuradha K, Jethwani P. Handbook on Inflammatory Bowel Disease (Volume 1). Hemakshee Publication. Sikar. 2024 ISBN: 978-81-969920-0-2

This book titled **"Handbook on Inflammatory Bowel Disease (Volume 1)"** is primarily intended to be a collection of peer reviewed and plagiarism free chapters written by research scholars, academicians, scientists, doctors and faculty members of their respective fields. Chapters of this book particularly based on topics such as etiology differential diagnosis, prevention and treatment of inflammatory bowel disease (IBD); malnutrition and IBD, role of yoga & meditation in IBD, yoga techniques & quality of life in patients with IBD, role of diet in IBD, use of micro-organisms in prevention & treatment of IBD, role of remission dict in IBD and pediatric IBD compass.

Note: These books are available on publisher's website, Amazon and FlipKart

www.ingramcontent.com/pod-product-compliance
Lightning Source LLC
LaVergne TN
LVHW010528200726
843506LV00013B/2740